1984

Organization of Medical Record Departments in Hospitals

Margaret Flettre Skurka

Mary E. Converse, Editor

American Hospital Publishing, Inc.

a wholly owned subsidiary of the American Hospital Association

Library of Congress Cataloging in Publication Data

Skurka, Margaret F.
    Organization of medical record departments in hospitals.

    Includes index.
    1. Medical records—Management. 2. Information storage
and retrieval systems—Hospitals. I. Converse, Mary E.
II. Title. [DNLM: 1. Medical records. 2. Hospital
departments—Organization and administration. WX 173 S629o]
RA976.S57 1983   658.5'04261   83-21535
ISBN 0-87258-344-9

Catalog no. 148151

© 1984 by
American Hospital Publishing, Inc.
211 East Chicago Avenue
Chicago, Illinois 60611

Printed in the U.S.A.
3M-12 / 83-001

Cover design by George Perry,
Star Publications, Chicago Heights, Illinois

Contents

iii

List of Figures

Preface

Recognizing hospitals' need for guidelines in developing efficient medical record systems and procedures, the American Hospital Association has published *Organization of Medical Record Departments in Hospitals.* This book is a revised edition and replacement of *Medical Record Departments in Hospitals: Guide to Organization,* published by the AHA in 1972. It marks the third edition of this publication; the first edition was published in 1962.

This book is designed to assist the hospital administrator and the individual in charge of medical records, particularly in small hospitals, in applying basic principles of medical record management in the establishment and ongoing review of the hospital's medical record system. Because appropriate application of these basic principles requires careful analysis of the individual hospital's needs, various methods and the advantages and disadvantages of each are presented.

Throughout the book, the use of the term *medical record practitioner* encompasses both the registered record administrator and the accredited record technician, because both levels hold a wide variety of positions within the medical record profession.

Mary Converse, American Hospital Association senior staff specialist, Medical Records, and director, Central Office on ICD-9-CM, was the project director and editor. The text was written by Margaret Skurka, assistant professor and director, Medical Record Technology Program, Indiana University School of Medicine at IU Northwest, Gary, Indiana, and a member of the panel of accreditation surveyors of the American Medical Record Association. The book was reviewed by Marsha Ladenburger, R.N., M.H.A., director, AHA Division of Quality Control Management.

Members of the advisory panel were Peggy Campbell, R.R.A., director of medical records, St. Anne's Hospital, Chicago, Illinois; Jean Stauber,

R.R.A., DRG coordinator, Mercy Hospital, Moose Lake, Minnesota; Minnette Terlep, A.R.T., St. Joseph Hospital, Joliet, Illinois; and Roberta E. Thompson, A.R.T., medical record director, Perry Memorial Hospital, Princeton, Illinois.

Editorial services were provided in house by Christie Enman, editor, and Karen Downing, editorial assistant, under the direction of Marjorie E. Weissman, manager, Book Editorial Department, and Dorothy Saxner, vice-president, Books.

Chapter 1

Introduction

The term *medical record* implies physician involvement and supervision of the medical care provided to an individual. The term *health record* may refer to a medical record, a record of services provided by nonphysician health practitioners, or a record of an individual's health status on file in an agency, insurance carrier's office, non-health-care institution, or other organization that is used in health benefits plans, applications for insurance, employment records, or references for development of social plans for individual or family care. Throughout this book, the term *medical record* rather than *health record* is used, because the book's primary focus is on the health records used and maintained in health care institutions, primarily hospitals.

Hospitals, ambulatory care facilities, emergency centers, trauma centers, rehabilitation and mental health centers or institutions, home care programs, and skilled nursing homes are classified as health care institutions. Health care institutions are characterized by having permanent facilities, providing medical or health care services to individuals, and maintaining medical records on every recipient of those services. Although health care institutions vary according to the type and range of medical and health-related services they provide, they all have a common need to concentrate within a given record all patient care information about an individual. Such concentration of information promotes communication among the staff directly involved in the patient's care, accuracy of significant information, continuity of patient care, and economy in record system management.

Another need common to all health care institutions is a medical record department that is organized and staffed to provide adequate record management systems and practices to facilitate use of the medical record while safeguarding the content from unauthorized disclosures. Allocation of resources necessary to the development and maintenance of a medical record department for maximum performance can greatly minimize duplication of recordkeeping and indexing by other departments or units within the institution.

The functions of the medical record department are service-oriented and support the optimal standards set forth for quality of care and services in the health care institution. Although the functions of and demands for services from the medical record department may vary according to the type of institution, the common denominator among all medical record departments is the maintenance of record systems in one or more forms to provide storage and ready retrieval of clinical information by patient name or number, physician name or number, diagnosis, procedure, and other subject items deemed necessary. The forms that medical records take are hard copy, miniaturized (microfilmed), or computer-assisted. Departmental functions are those activities that support current and continuing patient care, the administrative affairs of the institution, continuing education programs, health services research, patient accounts, utilization / risk management / quality assurance programs, legal and quasi-legal requirements, and extraneous patient services.

In the ensuing chapters of this book, the term *hospital* rather than health care institution is used for purposes of simplification and primary thrust.

Bylaws, rules, and regulations of the organized medical staff include principles and procedures governing an individual medical staff member's responsibility for maintaining timely, accurate, and complete medical records. The rules and regulations for medical records are applicable to the whole medical staff and should be evenly enforced. In keeping with the Joint Commission on Accreditation of Hospitals (JCAH) standards for rules and regulations to be adopted, the medical staff is responsible for:

- Approving the symbols and abbreviations that may be used in the medical record, determining when an explanatory legend is required on a medical record form, and disseminating the list of approved symbols and abbreviations to all members of the medical staff and appropriate members of the hospital staff
- Identifying the specific categories of hospital and medical personnel who are qualified to accept and transcribe verbal physician orders and when countersignatures on transcribed verbal orders are required
- Stating the amount of time following admission of the patient during which a history and physical examination must be entered in the medical record
- Issuing specific time limits for completion of medical records following patient discharge
- Requiring all entries in the medical record to be dated and authenticated by the responsible practitioner

The responsibility of the medical staff for the preceding medical record requirements does not end with adoption of written rules and regulations. There must be a mechanism for regular review and monitoring for compliance. This activity may be carried out by the medical staff as a whole in hospitals with small nondepartmentalized medical staffs, or it may be performed by a specific committee or by each department in larger hospitals with organized clinical services. Regardless of the mechanism used, medical records must be reviewed no fewer than four times a year for their timely completion, clinical pertinence, and overall adequacy. Such review is to include a sufficient sampling of inpatient, ambulatory care, emergency, and hospital-administered home care program medical records.

In addition to medical staff representation, the medical record review process should include participation of medical record personnel, nursing service staff, and any other professional personnel directly involved in medical record documentation. The objective is to evaluate the medical record for assurance that it includes sufficient documentation of the patient's condition, progress, and outcome of care; that there is documentary evidence of tests and therapy as ordered; and that there is documentation of notification and acceptance in any transfer of patient responsibility from one physician or dentist to another. The review process should take into consideration the adequacy of the medical record for hospitalwide quality assurance, utilization management, and risk management activities.

The responsibility of the organized medical staff for the patient medical records maintained by the hospital includes active participation in determining the format of the completed medical record, in approving the design of record forms, and in determining how the records will be preserved (hard copy, microfilm, or computer-assisted).

The CEO and the organized medical staff have an interdependent responsibility for enforcing completion of medical records. This is in keeping with the medical staff's bylaws, rules, and regulations for self-government, which are approved by the hospital's governing board. The medical record practitioner has responsibility for complying with the established rules and regulations for medical records and for reporting any deficiencies or violations to the CEO and the designated officer or committee of the medical staff. The working relationship between the medical staff and the medical record practitioner should include the development of services and procedures to facilitate completion of medical records.

Relationship of Physicians to Medical Records

The granting of staff membership and clinical privileges to a physician or a dentist by the organized medical staff makes that physician or dentist responsible for adhering to the medical staff's existing rules and regulations for medical records. When each member of the medical staff is reappraised

3

for reappointment to the medical staff, one of the items considered is the individual's maintenance of timely, accurate, and complete medical records. Physicians who serve as chiefs or directors of diagnostic or therapeutic departments or services are responsible for the timeliness, accuracy, and completeness of reports generated by them or their staff for inclusion in the medical record.

The clinical privileges accorded dentists and oral surgeons should delineate their responsibility for documenting procedure and diagnosis, writing orders, prescribing medications, and securing the physician's documentation of history, physical examination, and any medical problems. The qualifications of an oral surgeon will determine whether or not clinical privileges include documentation by the oral surgeon of the admission history, physical examination, and assessment of medical risks.

Clinical privileges granted to podiatrists include delineation of hospital admission privileges, such as a dual responsibility of the podiatrist and a physician member of the medical staff for patient care, the scope and extent of surgical procedures that may be performed by the podiatrist, and the authority of the podiatrist in writing orders and prescribing medications. The podiatrist is responsible for documentation of history and physical examination related to podiatry, procedure performed, and podiatry diagnosis. The attending physician is responsible for documenting the basic medical assessment of the patient and any medical problems.

Likewise, clinical privileges granted to other nonphysician professionals (psychologists, nurse practitioners, and so forth) must include delineation of their responsibility for medical record documentation and of any requirements for documentation and countersignatures by a physician member of the medical staff.

The rules and regulations of the medical staff and clinical departments delineate the authority and responsibility of house officers (interns and residents) for medical record documentation and the requirements for countersignatures or documented evidence of supervision and participation of the responsible attending physician in the care given the patient. The responsible attending physician may countersign the house officer's pertinent entries, or the attending physician may prefer to make separate entries in the medical record.

When the medical staff has approved a professional personnel category for such duties as taking medical histories and documenting some aspects of a physical examination, such entries in the medical record must be appropriately authenticated by the responsible physician or dentist.

The parts of the medical record that are the responsibility of the attending physician must be authenticated by that physician. This includes signing and dating the entries made by the physician and countersigning any entries made on behalf of the attending physician in lieu of an entry indicating the attending physician's concurrence or separate findings and judgments.

When rubber-stamp signatures are authorized for use in authenticating entries in the medical record, their use must be controlled. An individual whose signature a stamp represents is obligated to provide the CEO with a signed statement that only he or she has the stamp and is the only one who will use it. Pathologists and radiologists, for example, may prefer to use rubber stamps in authenticating their reports of findings and diagnoses or impressions.

The quality of the medical record depends on the timeliness and informational content entered by all individuals given the right and responsibility for documenting their participation in patient care. Hospital and medical staff policies determine who has the right and responsibility for documentation in the medical record. Usefulness of the medical record depends in part on the legibility of entries and on the ability to identify the individuals and their qualifications (titles) who have entered the information. Poor penmanship, poor forms design, or a combination of both may create problems in using the medical record for continuing patient care, abstracting data, and reviewing untoward incidents.

Relationship of the Governing Board to Medical Records

The governing board has the overall responsibility for the conduct of the hospital in making available high-quality patient care. Included in this responsibility is corporate planning to meet the health care needs of the community the hospital serves. To carry out its responsibilities, the governing board establishes mechanisms for fulfilling the necessary policymaking, planning, and administrative functions. This is done through establishing committees, appointing a chief executive officer, and making the medical staff a self-governing body.

The governing board holds the medical staff responsible for developing, adopting, and implementing bylaws, rules, and regulations by which it can govern itself. These bylaws, rules, and regulations include provisions for adequacy of medical records and are subject to the approval of the governing board before implementation.

The governing board appoints the CEO and holds the CEO responsible for implementing established policies in the operation of the hospital and for keeping the governing board well informed on hospital operations. The CEO is also responsible for informing the governing board of federal, state, and local affairs that may affect hospital operations and planning.

Although there is daily interaction between the CEO and members of the medical staff, there are liaison functions that require the combined efforts of the medical staff, the CEO, and the governing board. This is accomplished through establishing a joint committee to address activities of mutual concern.

Relationship of the CEO to Medical Records

The CEO's responsibility for medical records relates to ownership and services. The medical record is regarded as the property of the hospital and is maintained for the benefit of the patient, the medical staff, and the hospital. The CEO is responsible to the governing board for implementing a system for maintaining medical records on every individual who is evaluated or treated as an inpatient, ambulatory care patient, emergency patient, or patient who receives services in a hospital-administered home care program. The CEO also bears responsibility for safeguarding medical records against loss, defacement, tampering, unauthorized use of information contained therein, and fire and water damage.

The CEO is accountable for organizing the administrative functions of the hospital, delegating duties, and delineating and clarifying accountability for subordinates. This realm of responsibility includes providing a medical record department or service with a qualified manager and adequate staffing, equipment, space, and facilities to perform the functions required.

The person employed by the CEO to direct medical record department operations should be qualified by both education and administrative experience to organize and manage the hospital's medical record system. This individual must be able to work harmoniously and effectively with medical staff members, committees of the medical staff and the hospital, administrative and financial management staff members, and other department directors. The director of medical records should have middle-management skills in working with employees and in sharing responsibilities for hospitalwide programs. The duties of the department director should be clearly defined and his or her authority should be commensurate with the designated responsibilities.

The CEO should expect the medical record department director to be aware of medical record requirements related to hospital compliance with laws, regulations, and accreditation standards. However, hospital compliance will at times require intervention by the CEO to enforce hospital and medical staff rules and regulations on the completion, accessibility, and authorized uses of the medical records. Without such support, the department director may find it difficult or impossible to provide high-quality services and desired productivity standards.

Relationship of the Medical Record Practitioner to Medical Records

The medical record practitioner, whether serving as director of the department or supervisor of a section, performs duties in support of high-quality patient care. Providing services on a day-to-day basis and planning for future services and systems are based on the need to document the patient care provided by the hospital and the medical staff for the community served.

Depending on the size and scope of functions to be performed in the medical record department, qualifications for the department director may include being a registered record administrator or an accredited record technician. The director should have at least the documented equivalent in education and training of a medical record administrator or medical record technician.

The managerial skills of the department director must include ability to organize the functions and work load for maximum productivity; to provide overall directions to department personnel; to assist the medical staff in carrying out its responsibilities for timely, accurate, and complete medical records; to assist with and participate where appropriate in committee activities; and to adhere to the established policies, rules, and regulations of the hospital.

In small hospitals, the medical record practitioner may provide secretarial support services to medical staff activities, such as those activities carried out by a committee of the whole. The medical record practitioner who is knowledgeable about current JCAH standards, applicable state and federal regulatory requirements, and pertinent reference articles on medical staff activities can provide valuable assistance to small medical staffs. In any event, it is important that the medical record practitioner be regarded as a valuable resource person for medical staff activities. A practitioner should make information available and should draw attention to relevant points without giving the appearance of trying to direct activity.

The director of the medical record department must be aware of the working relationship between the hospital administration and the self-governing medical staff and the authority granted to each by the governing board. The department director will receive directions from both the administration and the medical staff, and at times their interests may conflict. It is important that the director maintain good working relationships with both. It may be necessary to coordinate their directives or to develop alternate proposals that will serve the best interests of both. The director should make an effort to avoid creating unnecessary differences between hospital administration and the medical staff.

The medical record practitioner will interact with all departments or services generating information for inclusion in the individual patient's medical record. The medical record practitioner should be familiar with the reporting systems and procedures used for generating reports in the diagnostic and therapeutic areas. The talents of the medical record practitioner should not be limited to record systems for the medical record department only. The medical record practitioner can also serve as a consultant or resource person for record systems in other areas of the hospital.

Delays in getting reports into patient medical records should be investigated to determine whether each delay is temporary or chronic, and the CEO or a designee should be advised of any problems. Missing records and late reports create delays in the completion of medical records and in the continuing care of the patient. Often, the medical record department is unjustly held accountable for this situation. Therefore, it behooves the director of the medical record department to maintain surveillance and take early action to avoid delays. It is important that all medical record practitioners maintain good communication and working relationships with other hospital departments and services. Admitting, data processing, social service, dietary, nursing, purchasing, and financial management must not be overlooked in strengthening communication for effective operations.

Of particular importance is the working relationship with the patient accounts or business office. The mechanisms now used to process bills for payment of hospital services include a report on diagnostic and procedural information. More and more emphasis is being placed on the accuracy and completeness of the statements and codes for diagnoses and operations. Very few business office personnel possess the skills or knowledge to report diagnostic and procedural data as accurately or completely as medical record personnel who have had training and experience in abstracting and coding. Therefore, medical record practitioners have or will become involved in providing the clinical data necessary to process claims within 24 to 48 hours after patient discharge.

Adding the abstracting and coding function of claims processing to the medical record department may require reorganizing priorities and work assignments to provide the clinical data on a timely basis. It may also require initiatives in communicating with members of the medical staff the hospital's need for immediate completion of a discharge summary form at the time of each patient's discharge.

The medical record practitioner's sense of success and accomplishment can often be related to the immediate availability and the high usage rate of medical records within the hospital. Medical records are viable tools for patient care, health services statistics, substantiation of patient care services and treatment provided, continuing education programs, health services and clinical research, quality assurance, and risk management.

Chapter 2

Location, Space, and Equipment Requirements

The value of the medical record and the operational concept of medical record services are important considerations in determining location and space requirements. In planning or deciding location and space allocation, key considerations and questions include the following:

- What hospital services are the responsibility of the medical record department?
- How will records and notices flow to and from the admitting department, nurses' stations, emergency department, clinics, business office, and so forth?
- How will all reports of diagnostic tests and other notations be added to the record or delivered to the medical record department?
- Will records of readmitted patients be sent automatically to the nursing unit or will physicians come to the medical record department for them?
- Will physicians complete medical records in the medical record department or in some other area of the hospital?
- Who will be authorized access to medical records and the master patient index if the department is not staffed 24 hours a day, 7 days a week?
- Will ambulatory care and emergency care records be filed in the medical record department? If so, will there be an integrated record to establish a unit record system?
- What numbering system is to be used, unit or serial, and will the terminal-digit filing system be used?
- Will filing equipment be open-shelf or will it be the high-density type? Will an electronic filing, storage, and retrieval system be used?
- What is the preservation period for medical records? How long will medical records be retained in active files within the department? Will

9

inactive records be retained in hard copy and, if so, where will they be filed? Will inactive medical records be stored on microfilm?

- Are there plans to use automated equipment or computer-assisted systems that will increase or decrease space needs?
- Will abstracting and coding of medical records for indexes and collection and processing of statistical data include inpatients and ambulatory care, emergency, and home care patients?
- What is the extent of data abstracting and coding for hospitalwide programs such as quality assurance, utilization management, and risk management?
- How many requests are received for release of medical record information to sources outside the hospital in the form of letters, telephone calls, and subpoenas or court orders?
- How much statistical reporting is carried out in the medical record department?
- Will the medical record department have any responsibility for the medical staff library?

Location

Continuous communication exists between the medical record department and the admitting departments in the inpatient, ambulatory care, and emergency care units. In addition, the medical record department must communicate clinical information and codes to the business office for claims processing and receive notices of discharges and reports of diagnostic and therapeutic procedures. Throughout each day, a large percentage of members of the medical staff will be completing or referencing medical records in the department. To ensure prompt completion of and ready access to medical records, it is advisable that the medical record department be located along the pathway most often used by physicians and near the admitting department, emergency department, and business office. If the medical record department is not staffed 24 hours a day, it should be located within easy walking distance of admitting or nursing staff authorized to reference files and retrieve records on an emergency basis. The need for security surveillance to safeguard medical record information and equipment during hours in which the department is closed should also be considered.

Space Requirements

Space allocation is determined by departmental services to be provided, equipment and systems to be used, and daily work load. Although services may vary somewhat from hospital to hospital, services and tasks to be considered in allocating space include the following.

Record File Maintenance

Record file maintenance includes retrieving, dispatching, receiving, and filing of records in active and, to a lesser degree, in inactive files. Open-shelf filing equipment may be 8 shelves or 10 shelves high. A 36-inch open shelf can house approximately 75 average inpatient records or 300 average outpatient or emergency records. High-density open-shelf filing allows filing units to be electrically operated for access and takes less space than other open-shelf filing units. If a unit-numbering system is used, adequate space must be provided on the shelf for growth of records as a result of readmissions and repeat clinic visits. A review of records from the past several years is the best source of information for working estimates of the amount of space required. One approach is to tabulate the average number of sheets per medical record of discharged patients over two or three months, counting the sheets per current episode of care plus the sheets per previous episode of inpatient or outpatient care. This tabulation provides the size of an average medical record.

The terms *active* and *inactive* are used to refer to both medical records and file locations. A medical record is classified as active when the last discharge or visit date is within three to five years of the current date. Active records are maintained in readily accessible files, referred to as *active files*. If there is a sharp decline in readmissions between three and five years, the active file space may need to accommodate records for only three years.

Statistical data should be maintained on the rate of readmissions to assist in planning for current and future space needs and to provide information for use in department and hospital administration. A count of readmissions within 1 month, 3 months, 6 months, 1 year, 2 years, 3 years, 5 years, and 10 or more years from date of last discharge would be helpful for multiple purposes. The utilization management program may be interested in data on readmissions within 1 to 6 months of the latest discharge.

Inactive records are less often retrieved and filed. *Inactive files* may be located in an area that is not as quickly accessible as that for active files. Inactive records are often microfilmed to save space by miniaturization. Microfilming also provides easy accessibility. Space allocation for microfilmed records includes space for the storage container, viewer, copier, and any camera equipment used for in-house filming. The length of time medical records must be retained in original or microfilm form varies from state to state. Each state hospital association can provide the necessary information on legal requirements for the retention of medical records (inpatient and outpatient). The Healthcare Financial Management Association publishes a handbook entitled *Guide to the Retention and Preservation of Records with Destruction Schedules*, which contains one section devoted to state regulations and recommended retention period for various types of hospital clinical records. See also the AHA Technical Advisory Bulletin *Preservation of Medical Records in Health Care Institutions.*

Master Patient Index

Space allocation for the master patient index will depend on the type of equipment or system used for immediate identification of current and past patients by name, address, birthdate, and medical record number at a minimum. This information may be stored on 1½-inch by 3-inch or 3-inch by 5-inch cards in upright cabinets or in electrical rotary files, or it may be stored in a computer-assisted system with terminals to access the file. The master patient index is maintained as a permanent record and, when necessary, names may be culled by age or birthdate for inactive storage. Efficiency dictates that inactive storage be located near the active files for rapid retrieval of records as needed for patient care purposes.

Discharge Analysis

Desk or table space is needed to assemble current discharge records in permanent filing format, check for record completeness, initiate incomplete record follow-up notices, and fill out other forms as necessary.

Disease and Operative Index and Statistical Data

Desk space that will accommodate medical records, coding books, reference books, and abstract forms is needed for compiling disease and operative indexes and statistical data. If a manual system is used, filing equipment for the indexes will be necessary. If an automated data processing mechanism is used, terminals or miniprocessing equipment must be accommodated on or next to the desk.

Correspondence

Space for desks, telephones, typewriters, and duplicating equipment is necessary for handling telephone calls and written requests for disclosure of medical record information.

Word Processing

The space needed for word processing will be determined by size of the typewriter desk, plus the type of equipment used for dictation and transcription of clinical reports and summaries.

Administration

The manager of the department should have an office with sufficient space for supervisory meetings and private conversations.

Record Completion

Desk or table space with provision for private dictation must be provided for members of the medical staff to complete their patients' medical records.

In addition, space must be provided for review, study, and abstracting of records as needed for medical staff activities and for bona fide study or research. Bookcases or shelves may be needed to temporarily house the medical records pending use in this area.

Other Requirements

In addition to the space required for the services already mentioned, a small work area with a table is needed for use by lawyers, insurance representatives, and others who are authorized to read a particular medical record. This area should be separate from the physician work area.

Carts for transporting records, bins or tables for sorting medical records, and bookcases or shelves for reference materials and supplies will be needed. Employee lockers may be placed inside or outside the department.

Because file cabinets occupy more space than upright shelving, their use should be kept to a minimum. Two sections of double-faced open shelves occupy approximately 12 square feet of floor space, whereas nine five-drawer file cabinets occupy approximately 26 square feet of floor space. Both arrangements accommodate approximately 1,100 letter-size filing inches.

Electric typewriters are the mainstay of the medical record department and should be selected according to the tasks to be performed. An executive typewriter may be needed to prepare official committee minutes and reports. Typewriters with continuous feed and timesaving features merit use in word processing and in preparing patient index cards.

Occupational Safety and Health Act (OSHA) standards for space determinations designate that secondary aisles be a minimum of three feet wide and that main thoroughfares be at least five feet wide.

To provide adequate work space, 60 square feet per employee is suggested for desk arrangements. When the ideal configuration and space allocation are not available, the department director must resort to innovative ideas for furniture and equipment selection. The manager must be familiar with principles of layout and functional planning to design the work space for maximum operational efficiency.

Work Load

The work load of the medical record department is an important determinant of space and equipment requirements. Work load levels are based on the volume of materials being processed on a daily, weekly, monthly, and yearly basis. The amount of material being processed per day, week, or month in each of the service areas of the department should be determined, including the number of new admissions added to the master patient index and how many times this index is used; the number of discharges processed; the number of lines of typed material generated in transcription; the number of requests for release of medical record information; the number of records being abstracted and coded and the number of items of data this entails; the number of records being retrieved, dispatched, and refiled; and any expected changes in work loads. The work load figures obtained for one year can change in the next year if the hospital's corporate planning includes additional patient care facilities. Therefore, it may be necessary to project future work loads when planning for space and equipment.

Space limitations caused by an increase in the work load may require operating one or more service areas 16 or 24 hours per day. In large hospitals, three or more department service areas may be in operation 24 hours a day, 7 days a week.

Systems and Equipment

The department director should aim toward the use of the best methods for generation and flow of medical record information and the selection of products that meet the hospital's need for efficient production and high quality at reasonable cost. Before equipment and systems are selected, the features to be assessed should be itemized, including the following:

- Will this system or equipment meet the needs of current and projected work loads?
- Will additional space be needed if the work load increases?
- Will paperwork be reduced and, if so, by what percentage?
- Can information or data be changed or updated easily and quickly?
- Does the system or equipment have the necessary flexibility for integration with other systems or equipment in the department and hospital?
- Can this system or equipment perform a variety of tasks or applications?
- How much space does it require?
- Is this system or equipment cost-effective from the standpoint of reduced personnel time or increased productivity?
- What are the warranty period and provisions, the costs for various types of maintenance, and the response time for service calls?
- Is a backup system needed for down time?
- What is the amount of training time needed for employees? Will the vendor provide training? Is training material available?
- Will the vendor provide support services in the development of applications? If so, is there any cost associated with it?
- What is the reputation of the vendor or the vendor's company? Will the company provide references for an overall evaluation of system, equipment, or services?
- What is the purchase price? Is leasing or rental an optional feature?

Technological changes are occurring at a rapid rate, and equipment and systems offer new and improved features every year. Often, the basic decision to be made is whether a task to be performed is best served by a standalone mechanical or electronic system or by a shared or integrated computer-based system.

In general, equipment needs for the individual hospital medical record department are affected by:

- Work schedule and work week, which may allow certain types of equipment to be used over long periods and may require a good communication and dispatch system for skeleton staff coverage of the master patient index and file room during evening and weekend hours.
- A decentralized medical record system for inpatient and outpatient records or a separate location for word processing, which may require transport and communication systems and equipment.
- Number of visits to the emergency service and clinics, which require STAT requests for medical records, and the number of scheduled visits to the clinics, which require medical records to be retrieved and dispatched before clinic hours. All of these may require electronic or computer-assisted systems for record requests and sign-out.
- Statistical data needs, which require mechanization of data processing and investigation of the possibility of a data base integrated with the business office system or main computer system.
- Paperwork and duplication of data entries that could be reduced by use of computer terminals, miniprocessors, and encoding equipment that converts natural language to disease and procedure classification codes.

Support Areas

The medical record department, like other departments in the hospital, needs access to classrooms or meeting rooms for conducting in-service training programs and staff meetings. Provisions should be made to allow the medical record department to schedule use of this space. The services of the hospital's in-service education and training program should also be made available to the medical record department.

Chapter 3

Unit Record, Numbering, and Filing Systems

Maintaining an account of all patient care services provided to each patient, identification of the patient and the patient's medical record, and ready retrieval of the record are essential parts of a hospital medical record system. More specifically, efficient operation of the medical record department depends on the design and interaction of tasks to:

- Merge and preserve the documentation of patient care provided by various professional services to an individual during an episode of care
- Merge or cross-reference records of patient care provided to an individual during more than one episode of care
- Identify each patient and that patient's medical record by a unique number
- Provide a designated filing location of each patient's medical record
- Account in writing for removal of any record from its filing location

Various methods are used in designing task-oriented systems for the medical record department. The method chosen depends on the types of patient care services provided by the hospital, the annual rate of admissions and visits, the availability of automated or mechanized equipment, and department space allocation. The common goal among all medical record departments is efficiency and accuracy in the maintenance of chronological record, numbering, and filing systems.

Unit Record

The unit record is a single chronological record that documents the medical care provided to an individual during stays in the hospital, visits to the ambulatory care and emergency departments, and hospital-sponsored home care.

17

A chronological record is an arrangement of patient care information in the order of occurrence of events and findings. The principle of chronological arrangement in a medical record pertains to a single episode of care as well as to multiple episodes of care as an inpatient or outpatient. For example, after discharge of an inpatient, the medical record sheets for that stay in the hospital are assembled in chronological order for physician entries, diagnostic reports, and nursing entries; the visits of patients to the ambulatory care or emergency facilities are arranged in chronological order; and the visits of staff members to a home care patient are arranged in chronological order. When a patient has had more than one episode of care as an inpatient or outpatient, a chronological record is maintained by incorporating and arranging these episodes by dates. An exception to the chronological unit record is exclusion of test reports, such as results of clinical laboratory tests generated on private outpatient referrals, for which the site of care remains the physician's office (generally referred to as private outpatient referrals for tests only).

When feasible, the unit record should include documentation of hospital-sponsored home care. For home care patients, the unit record would be held in the home care office for timely updating and reference, but it must be readily accessible for use in clinic or emergency service visits and hospital admissions. Hospital stays followed by continuing care in the hospital's ambulatory care facility or home care program present problems in record completion, filing of loose reports, abstracting, and coding. However, the value of the unit record for patient care and study purposes must be weighed against the extra costs in the personnel time and the equipment needed to track the unit record location at all times and to retrieve and dispatch records as needed. Also, each member of the hospital and medical staff involved in the use of the unit record must be aware of and sensitive to the need for ready accessibility of the record at all times.

The unit record is maintained to provide members of the staff with necessary references to a patient's current and past conditions, procedures performed, and patient's response to therapy. As such, the unit record cannot remain in the domain of any one staff member or patient care area. The medical record department must be able to exercise authority in retrieving the medical record from any location for purposes of patient care. At times, it may be necessary for the CEO to provide the department head with necessary backup in enforcing medical record accessibility.

A hospital may contract for outside services, such as for certain clinical laboratory tests or for pathology services. The reports prepared by these outside services are filed as a part of the patient's medical record. Approval by the organized medical staff and the CEO is necessary before copies of laboratory and x-ray reports from the private physician's office can be filed in the hospital medical record as a substitute for reports generated on an inpatient. If the hospital contracts for outside professional services, such as for physical therapy, the report of therapy given and the patient's progress must be entered into the individual patient's hospital medical record. When physician services are contracted for to provide emergency service care, the original report of findings, care given, and disposition of the patient are filed in the hospital medical record. The emergency service physician is entitled to a copy of the emergency service record.

The cost of maintaining a unit record system is offset by the elimination of or reduction in the maintenance of duplicate patient care records in various clinical and therapeutic departments.

Alternatives to the Unit Record

Hospitals that administer or sponsor freestanding ambulatory care facilities may not find the unit record system feasible. When it is not feasible to combine into a single record all documentation of inpatient, ambulatory, emergency, and home care, there must be a cross-referencing system to identify the patient and the patient's component medical records. A method must be devised for retrieval and availability of the patient's component medical records when the patient is admitted to the hospital or appears for an ambulatory care appointment. This can be accomplished through the use of a computer-assisted system that maintains an up-to-date integrated record of pertinent information. A computer-assisted system allows each patient care site access to information about the individual patient's current condition, findings, treatment given, and response to treatment. When computer capabilities are not available, a procedure should be established for incorporating copies of discharge summaries and diagnostic tests in ambulatory care and home care records. The inpatient records should also include summarized data on ambulatory care and home care services provided to the patient. The latter implies that ambulatory care and home care records will be available on the patient's admission to the hospital and will be summarized at that time or will be summarized and available in the event of scheduled hospital admissions.

Hospitals serving a transient population, such as those in a resort area, may have no need for a unit record system. However, for the permanent population the hospital does serve, a single record system should be maintained for each individual, perhaps by bringing together all inpatient records on each individual.

If the hospital does not have an ambulatory care service, a unit record is maintained by a single record of all stays in the hospital and all visits to the emergency department.

Format of the Unit Record

Members of the medical and hospital staff appointed to review the medical record function also are responsible for standardizing the format of the medical record. Usually, the format of the record maintained on the nursing unit is quite different from that of the record used for permanent filing. The standardized format should facilitate making entries, referencing material, reviewing the record for completeness, assessing the quality of care given, and abstracting for reporting and collecting statistical data. The type of folder used to house the medical record provides options such as the placement of ambulatory care records on the right side and inpatient records on the left side or vice versa. Folders with middle separations allow the parts of the medical record less frequently referenced, such as nurses' notes, to be placed separately, if this is deemed desirable. Consideration should be given to a prominently placed form designed for dating and listing all inpatient and outpatient diagnoses and surgical procedures. Such a form provides for a quick review plus rapid reference to a particular diagnosis. The standardized format for collating episodes of care usually places the most current period of care first.

A unit record of a patient with multiple admissions or a long period of ambulatory care may require more than one folder. When more than one folder is needed for a particular patient's record, it is important to number the folders and to identify the total number of folders issued. For example, a unit record could entail three folders, and the folders should be identified as volume 1 of 3 volumes, volume 2 of 3 volumes, and volume 3 of 3 volumes. Innovations that will simplify the recording, review, or timeliness of retrieval of information should be encouraged, without sacrificing the quality and basic content requirements.

Numbering Systems

In any large system involving the names of people, such as bank accounts, charge accounts, life or health insurance policies, and so forth, unique numbers are issued to differentiate one individual from another. The types of numbering systems include unit numbering, serial numbering, annual numbering, use of Social Security numbers, and family numbering.

Unit-Numbering System

A unit-numbering system is based on a one-time issue of a number to a patient. On all subsequent admissions or visits that same number is used to identify that patient and the patient's medical record. Excluded from the unit-numbering system are private outpatient admissions for tests only, such as for laboratory tests. It is possible to develop one unit-numbering system to serve a number of functions within the hospital. The development of a master index of names, maintained either by mechanized equipment or computer-assisted programs, to provide rapid and accurate identification, can be cost beneficial. It would allow one numbering system to be used to identify patient medical records, patient accounts, x-ray films, tracings, personnel health records, and the like.

When the unit-numbering system is used, admitting clerks in the emergency department, ambulatory care units, and inpatient care units must be able to determine within a few minutes whether or not a medical record number already exists for an individual patient. In lieu of a computerized system, the medical record department must be able to respond immediately to provide the necessary information. Provision must be made for issuing unit numbers as needed. This can be done by issuing biweekly or monthly a block of numbers or a batch of numbered folders to each admitting area for use in initiating new medical record numbers. A multiple-part admitting form can be designed to provide a completed patient index card for the medical record department that includes the unit-number assignment.

The maintenance of any number identification system requires written procedures for handling any errors made in number identification assignments. Clerical errors that can occur include the assignment of the same identification number to different patients, transposition of digits in copying the identification number, and the assignment of a new identification number to a patient who has one on file. The last type of error is usually best corrected after the patient's discharge. When corrections are made in patient-identification-number assignments, all departments and services involved in the diagnostic workup and treatment of the patient must be notified in writing of the change. The business office must also be notified. Steps for correcting identification number errors must be carefully worked out to prevent errors and delays in verification of patient identification, such as in the patient verification procedures used by laboratory and blood bank technologists and x-ray technicians.

The use of a unit-numbering system for medical records affects space allocations for filing records. Each shelf must be able to accommodate growth in the size of individual records due to readmissions and continued visits to ambulatory care clinics. In assigning a given number of medical records to each shelf file, allow 25 percent of the shelf space for future increases in the bulk of the records. Additional space per filing shelf will be available as medical records not used for three to five years are moved to the inactive file. However, in a unit-numbering system, both the unit number and the medical record are reactivated when the patient returns. During any year, a certain number of records will move from the inactive file to the active file.

The unit-numbering system requires more intense service and control by the medical record department than other systems, but it provides the basis for integration of inpatient, ambulatory care, emergency department, and home care records.

Serial-Numbering System

The serial-numbering system provides a new identification number for each individual patient and the patient's medical record for each stay in the hospital and for each episode of ambulatory or emergency service care. The serial-numbering system is more suitable for use in hospitals that do not have ambulatory care facilities than for those that do.

The serial-numbering system is compatible with a unit record system for inpatient medical records. Each time the patient is admitted, all previous inpatient records are brought forward and filed under the latest identification number issued to the patient. The system requires a cross-referencing system for number identification in the master patient index and in the medical record files. All serial identification numbers assigned to a particular patient must be listed under the patient's name in the master patient index. As records are removed from their filing location, a cross-reference note to the latest identification number must be made. In hospitals with frequent readmissions, the medical record numbers must be continually updated, index cards must be changed to designate the most recently assigned identification number, and medical record files must be guided to the current filing location of previous records.

If the hospital has an ambulatory care program, the serial-numbering system will not be effective in integrating inpatient and outpatient medical records. Ambulatory care records cannot be assigned new identification numbers on each visit without disruption of both patient care and an ongoing medical record. When inpatient and outpatient medical record systems are maintained separately, the identification numbers can be cross-referenced at the time of admission to the hospital. However, some means must be established to distinguish between the two numbering systems. The year of registration in the ambulatory care program, followed by the serial registration number, is one means of differentiating the two numbering systems. The year of registration in the identification number makes it easy to spot records that may be candidates for transfer from active to inactive files.

The continued use of the serial-numbering system in hospitals with active ambulatory care programs should be assessed on the basis of failure to reach the goals of an integrated (unit) medical record system, time expended and expense incurred in maintaining the serial unit number system or two numbering systems, the number of reports misfiled and the impact of these errors on patient care, difficulties and delays created by lack of reference to the most current identification number in various indexes and secondary files, and backlogs in updating the active files.

Other Numbering Systems

Other types of numbering systems sometimes used by hospitals are the annual-numbering system, Social Security numbers, and the family-numbering system.

Serial numbering that includes the last two digits of the current calendar year may be used by hospitals that serve primarily a transient population.

The two digits for the year are added to the end of a serial number. The year designation serves as a control number in retiring inactive records. Also, the serial number plus the calendar year provides immediate data on the number of hospital admissions or visits during the year.

The Social Security number is a unique identification number and is collected when patients eligible for Medicare benefits are admitted. The number is used in the hospital billing mechanism for identification of Medicare patients. From the standpoint of logistics and personal privacy rights, the use of an individual's Social Security number to identify both the patient and the patient's medical record is discouraged.

It is important that the hospital have control of its patient identification numbering system. The hospital has no control over the Social Security numbering system, and it does not have access to the Social Security Administration files to verify a patient's name and Social Security number. With the exception of Medicare recipients, a patient may provide different Social Security numbers, and the hospital has no way of verifying whether or not any of the Social Security numbers given have been assigned to that individual by the Social Security Administration.

The Social Security number may not be available at the time of a patient's admission or visit, and the patient has the right to withhold the Social Security number without being denied care. In these instances, a separate numbering system or a pseudo-Social-Security numbering system must be used for patient identification. This results in the maintenance of two numbering systems. A pseudo-Social Security number could harm the patient, should the number be disclosed in authorized reports to third parties who assume it is the patient's real Social Security number. A pseudo-Social Security number can leave a trail that may take the patient years to unravel. If a patient's Social Security number is not available at the time of admission but is available later, the medical record department must then spend extra time and money to make the necessary changes in the medical record and in numerous indexes and files.

The 1977 report of the Privacy Protection Study Commission, entitled *Personal Privacy in an Information Society*, concludes that most opposition to the use of the Social Security number is directed at the record that would be created, as opposed to use of the number for personal identification. When an individual's records are identified by that individual's Social Security number, records or information about the individual could be exchanged, consolidated, and linked for purposes that may be unfair to the individual. Individuals may also resent being labeled with a number, especially with a Social Security number. The Commission further advised that any consideration of a standard universal label that could approximate a central population register and record system be postponed until society, through its legislatures, has made significant progress in establishing effective policies to regulate the use and disclosure of information about individuals collected by both private organizations and government agencies.

Family medicine programs may find it useful to identify individuals and their medical records by family association. In a family-numbering system, a unique number is assigned to the family, followed by a unique number to identify each member of the family. The family number is in reality a household number, because it includes only those indiviudals living within a given household. It includes grandparents, aunts, and uncles living in the household, but excludes family members who have moved away from the household. Therefore, the family number assignment may identify individuals who have different last names.

The medical record of the head of the household contains a complete health profile of each person living in the household. As each member of a given household enrolls for care in the family practice clinic, the medical record number assigned to that individual is based on the family number, to which a unique number to identify the individual family member is added. Not only does the family-numbering system support the concept of family practice, but it also provides a means of ready reference for health information on other members of the family that can be used in determining any patterns of illness or hereditary conditions that may occur within a family unit. The family-numbering system also provides a practical means for collection of statistical data, by household.

Filing Systems

Medical records can be filed using one of two types of filing systems, straight-numerical filing or terminal-digit filing.

Straight-Numerical Filing

The straight-numerical filing system is the arrangement of records by medical record identification numbers, starting with the lowest number and ending with the highest number. The highest numbers, which are the most recent, represent the greatest amount of retrieval and filing activity. Therefore, more activity and personnel will be concentrated in one part of the file area. Because this filing system does not disperse activity and personnel for maximum use of the entire file area, when records are pulled for clinic appointments or loose reports are filed with medical records, one part of the file area can become congested, and time can be lost in performing the tasks at hand.

Personnel are usually familiar with the principle of filing by number sequence; therefore, less in-service training is needed. However, quality controls are needed to ensure that records are filed correctly. Unless the entire medical record number is checked before the record is filed, it is possible to misfile it by a hundred or a thousand number sequence. Finding a misfile may also be more time-consuming in a straight numerical sequence file than in a terminal-digit file, in which colored folders may be used to enhance the accuracy of filing medical records.

Terminal-Digit Filing

Terminal-digit filing is a method that provides equal distribution of medical records in filing units throughout the file area. By providing an equal occupancy rate for shelving the records, terminal-digit filing also permits a more even work-flow pattern. File clerks retrieve and file records in all parts of the file area, rather than in just one part.

As the name implies, terminal-digit filing for medical records is based on the last two digits of the medical record number. For example:

The filing units could be divided into 100 sections, starting with 00 and ending with 99. A medical record label of 512640 would be read as 51-26-40, with the last two digits, 40, designating the first order of file location. All records ending in 40 would be located in a designated section. The second order of the filing arrangement is based on the middle two digits of the medical record number, 26. The medical record 51-26-40 would be filed behind a shelf guide labeled 26-40 along with all other records that have last digits of 2640. If five second-order divisions are allocated per filing shelf, the terminal-digit arrangement and sequence of medical records with the last four digits ranging from 2540 through 2940 would be as follows: First division 01-25-40, 02-25-40, 03-25-40, 04-25-40, 05-25-40, and so forth. Second division 01-26-40, 02-26-40, 03-26-40, 04-26-40, 05-26-40, and so forth. Third division 01-27-40, 02-27-40, 03-27-40, 04-27-40, 05-27-40, and so forth. Fourth division 01-28-40, 02-28-40, 03-28-40, 09-28-40, 10-28-40, and so forth. Fifth division 06-29-40, 07-29-40, 10-29-40, 11-29-40, 12-29-40, and so forth.

There are gaps in medical record numbers behind the divisions for 28 through 40 and 29 through 40. These gaps represent records that have been moved to the inactive files. Removal of inactive records does not alter the terminal-digit filing arrangement.

The key to a terminal-digit filing system is a design that permits clerks to visualize the actual location of the record in the file when reading the medical record number. The retrieval and filing time may be faster when the clerk is able to read 51-26-40 as: go to section 40, look behind guide 26, and retrieve (or file) record 51. In large file areas, the file room may be divided into stations, with a clerk assigned to each station. Station 1 would cover records with numbers ending in 00 through 19, station 2 would cover records with numbers ending in 20 through 29, station 3 would cover records with numbers ending in 30 through 39, and so forth.

When vertical shelf units are used and floor space is sufficient, the middle 5 shelves of an 8-shelf or 10-shelf unit can be used for active records and the remaining shelves used for inactive records. Various layouts should be considered to ensure maximal use of available file space. Medical records can be sorted before filing into terminal-digit filing order with the use of 10 bins or large trays. As medical records are returned for filing, they can be placed in the appropriate bins. For example, all records with numbers ending in 00 through 09 would be placed in one bin, those ending in 10 through 19 in another bin, and so forth. Such sorting procedures greatly facilitate the actual filing task.

The training period for terminal-digit filing may be a few hours longer than for conventional filing systems, but the overall advantages of the system compensate for the training time required.

Numbering Style

The method used for printing and writing the patient's identification number on forms, folders, and charge plates merits attention. It is common practice in many businesses to divide identification or account numbers into groups of two or three digits with a space or hyphen to accent the division. In some instances, a one-digit or two-digit division in a certain location within the number represents a code. In the terminal-digit filing system, the last two digits indicate the filing section and the filing unit. Dividing a four-digit to six-digit number into two-digit divisions (for example, 102040 would be written 10-20-40) promotes accuracy in reading and copying the number.

A basic method used in hospitals is to provide a three-part numbering style, 00-00-00. This provides a basis for uniformity, familiarity, and expansion. If this style is not in use, and if the highest number in present use is a five-digit number, such as 51234, it would be converted to read 05-12-34. All new forms and data systems in the hospital would automatically be designed to accommodate a six-digit number and would allow eight spaces for the identification number. When there is reason to start fresh in numbering, old numbers can be distinguished from the new numbers by using the following style, 00-00-01, 00-00-02, 00-00-03. The digital arrangement and the use of zeros to show the new style will differentiate between current number assignments and previously assigned numbers.

Color Coding

Medical record folders may be color coded to facilitate sorting and filing and to minimize misfiling problems. Color-coded folders were originally developed as part of a terminal-digit filing plan. A color scheme with designated color locations on the folder is used to identify the file location for the medical record number. A color coding scheme can be simple or detailed, depending on the needs of the individual hospital and on the cost of colored folders. Color-coded folders with already printed medical record numbers can be purchased from medical record form companies. The use of opaque coloring usually ensures obtaining the same color shade when record folders are reordered.

A do-it-yourself color coding scheme can be developed and implemented with the use of colored tape. X-ray departments often use color coded tape on film jackets to enhance filing accuracy or to code the latest date of the films within a jacket.

Record Charge-out and Tracking Methods

Methods selected for requisitioning medical records, charging out records, and tracking the location of records are just as important as the selection of numbering and filing systems and filing equipment. The medical record department is responsible for maintaining controls on records not in file.

The following should be considered in developing (or revising) methods for requisitioning and charging out records:

- Identification of a uniform data base for requisitioning and charging out that includes medical record number, patient's name, date of request, date record was dispatched to requester, name of person or clinic requesting record, name of person calling for record if different from that of the person requesting it, and location and telephone extension number within the hospital where the medical record will be used and located
- Establishment of a uniform size, such as 3 inches by 5 inches, for all requisition and charge-out forms
- The possibility of using a copy of the clinic appointment form as the requisition and charge-out form for records going to clinics
- Simplification of paperwork by designing multiple-part forms or pads with carbon inserts to provide one copy for use in the charge-out file and another copy to dispatch with the medical record
- Development of rules or guidelines for use by medical record personnel in knowing, by job title, which hospital staff members are authorized and not authorized to request records
- Selection of a plastic or other durable 4 inch by 13 inch (or larger if necessary) paddle with a clear plastic pocket for insertion of the charge-out slip
- Establishment of a medical record practice that any record not in its filing location, including the records of patients currently in the hospital, records being completed, and records being used within the medical record department, must be accounted for by an appropriate charge-out slip

With a few exceptions and some modifications, the above considerations can be used in developing a computer-assisted program for record charge-out and tracking. In departments that process 1,000 or more records in and

27

out of the files per day, optical scanning equipment may be used for documenting all record charge-outs and returns.

Loose Reports and Extraneous Matter

The principle of centralizing all information pertaining to an individual patient in a single record is encouraged, with few exceptions. Where feasible, copies of x-ray reports on private outpatient referrals should be incorporated into any existing hospital record on that patient. In this instance, the physician's office may receive the original report, since it is the site of patient care. Because the value of the results of laboratory tests performed on private outpatient referrals usually has a time limit, the cost involved in referencing the patient index for any existing hospital medical record and in filing the report may not justify efforts to centralize that information.

To provide a filing location and easy access, patient-identifiable correspondence and reports generated by outside parties may be filed in the medical record folder along with the patient's medical record, but should not be considered a part of the patient's medical record maintained by the hospital. This includes correspondence relative to a particular hospital patient from insurance carriers, government agencies, and other health care institutions. Summaries or reports of patient care provided by another health care institution are filed with the patient's medical record, but are not considered a part of the hospital-maintained medical record. A central location for various information on individual patients, such as the medical record folder, may benefit patient care and assist in carrying out the business of the medical staff and hospital.

Measures should be developed for incorporating all diagnostic reports in the appropriate patient medical records soon after they are received in the medical record department. These include reports on outpatients, as well as reports on patients recently discharged from inpatient units.

Chapter 4

Components of the Medical Record

Standards for the maintenance and for the adequacy of medical records are established by the Joint Commission on Accreditation of Hospitals (JCAH) as a part of its standards for hospital operations. Granting of hospital accreditation is based on substantial overall compliance with standards for hospital operations, including medical record services. Standards for medical record services are published in JCAH's *Accreditation Manual for Hospitals*. Hospital standards are revised periodically to reflect changes in the delivery of health care services and with advances in medical care. It is the responsibility of the medical record practitioner to keep abreast of the standards for medical record services published in the latest edition of the *Accreditation Manual for Hospitals*. Bulletins published by JCAH should be read for information pertinent to functions of the medical record department.

The principle on which JCAH standards for medical record services are based is "The hospital shall maintain medical records that are documented accurately and in a timely manner, that are readily accessible, and that permit prompt retrieval of information, including statistical data." An adequate medical record service incorporates all pertinent clinical information on a patient within a single record for current and continuing care purposes and for utilization management and quality assessment activities.

Medical Record Structure

Medical record information can be structured in three ways: the source-oriented medical record, the medical record that uses integrated progress notes, and the problem-oriented medical record.

Source-Oriented Medical Record

The traditional hospital medical record is basically structured by source and arranged chronologically. It is divided into sections according to who provides the documented data, that is, the medical staff and other health professionals. Thus, the sections are labeled according to the source, such as physician's notes, clinical laboratory and x-ray reports, social services' notes, nurses' notes and charts, and so forth. Within each section, the information is entered in chronological sequence. Conceptually, the physician integrates the data from the various sources by means of progress notes. The physician's progress notes should provide an assessment of existing problems, reasons for therapeutic decisions, and course of illness or stay in the hospital. When properly maintained, the source-oriented medical record should reflect the physician's direction of patient care, communication with others directly involved in the care of the patient, course of illness, and conclusions.

Critics of the source-oriented medical record often cite its lack of consistent organization. Pertinent information may be difficult to find because the record is bulky and because there is no index to specific subject matter.

Integrated Progress Notes

Integrated, or universal, progress notes use one standard form, on which all progress notes by physicians and other health care professionals are recorded. This system of chronological recording of progress notes pools data from various disciplines and stimulates improved patient care through shared knowledge.

The advantages of the integrated progress notes system are:
- A patient's progress can be determined quickly and logically by each professional sharing in the responsibility for care of the patient.
- It is unlikely that one professional will overlook the documentation made by another professional, because all the information is concentrated in one place. This also reduces the time spent by professionals in reviewing the record and encourages concise recording of all information.
- The number of specialized medical record forms may be reduced; therefore, the record bulk is reduced.
- The team concept among health professionals is encouraged.
- Progress notes are recorded promptly to maintain chronological sequence.
- Unwarranted destruction of significant observations made by nursing staff is prevented.

The disadvantages of the integrated progress notes system are:
- Only one individual can document or review progress notes at a given time.
- Special training sessions for concise and appropriate documentation by nonphysician professional staff are necessary.
- It may be difficult to identify the professional discipline of the recorders unless they sign their notes in full and identify their titles or departments.

- It is necessary to differentiate the attending physician's documentation. This can be accomplished by having physicians begin their notes at the outside margin of the form and all other disciplines indent their notes, or vice versa.
- Progress notes may occasionally appear to conflict when they are documented in proximity and represent the opinions of many health professionals. For example, nursing notes often relate to more than therapy.

Hospitals initiating the integrated progress notes system should plan the change carefully. A planning committee should be appointed, with representatives from each discipline as well as from the medical record department. The committee should:

- Outline the reasons for the conversion to the integrated system and list the advantages and disadvantages of the change.
- Develop a form for use in the integrated system.
- Identify the forms that will be superseded by the new form, such as physician's progress notes, nursing notes, respiratory therapy notes, and physical therapy progress notes. However, medication and treatment records, as well as graphic sheets, will continue to be kept separate from the universal progress notes.
- Develop guidelines for recording the kind of notes that are to be included in the integrated system, who has authority to write notes, how the individuals making entries will be identified, where the recording will be done, and how accessibility of the charts will be controlled.
- Develop plans for the initial orientation of staff members involved in the changeover and for subsequent orientation of new employees.
- Obtain final approval of the medical record committee, the medical staff, and the administration. Without the strong support of these individuals, the system is difficult to implement.

Problem-Oriented Medical Record

The problem-oriented medical record (POMR) was introduced in the late 1950s. It is a method of organizing clinical information by dividing the record into four sections—data base, problem list, initial plan, progress notes—and recording the information in a problem-oriented format. The POMR is a unique approach to the practice of medicine and to the recording of information. Structured to provide a total approach to patient care, the POMR enumerates patient problems, and progress notes, orders, and all other documentation are referenced to the particular problems they concern. Because this method allows all of the patient's problems, medical and otherwise, to be brought into relationship with one another, it may assist physicians in treating patients more effectively.

The initial component of a POMR is the data base, which is the documentation of patients' expressions of their problems in their own words. The data base includes present illness, past history, review of systems, family and social history, and a physical examination, which is a requirement for all records. All of the information gathered in the data base is used by all members of the health care team in the diagnosis and treatment of the patient.

The second component of the POMR, the problem list, is an enumeration of all problems the patient has, whether they are medical, family, work, or social. For example, a problem in the patient's family can be the basis for the patient's recent anxiety neuroses. Each problem is numbered, titled, and dated. If the problem is resolved at a later date, this is indicated and dated. The patient's list of problems is developed from the data base by the physician. Care should be taken that a condition that is suspected or is to be ruled out appears not as a problem but rather as a component of a plan.

The third part of the POMR is the initial plan. The physician indicates a plan for collecting further information, and for diagnostic or therapeutic treatment.

The fourth part of the POMR, the progress notes, documents the patient's progress relative to the physician's goals. Progress notes are written in the SOAP (subjective, objective, assessment, plan) format. The subjective statement includes the symptomatic complaints the patient voices that cannot necessarily be measured or strictly defined. The objective statements are measurable, observable entities, such as blood pressure, respirations, pulse rate, or the result of a laboratory test. The assessment is a statement of what is currently happening with the patient. It may indicate the present condition of the patient and any changes in this condition. The plan indicates the physician's course of action for the patient, and may include what must be done immediately or may include a long-term plan.

The POMR system allows a logical, structured, and complete compilation of information concerning the patient. In the POMR system all the documentation in the chart centers on the patient's particular problems and on the steps necessary to solve those problems. Avoiding the fragmentation that often results when the source-oriented approach to documentation is used, the POMR provides a structure for continuity of patient care. This method makes it easy for each member of the health care team to follow the patient's course of treatment, understand the method of treatment, and see for which problem a particular medication or test was ordered. The POMR helps the health care team understand the patient's problems, see the interrelationship of these problems, and decide the best way to proceed with treatment.

The POMR format may be advantageous in a teaching hospital, where many individuals document in the record and where the record can be initiated at the ambulatory care level and carried through inpatient care without fragmentation. It can be an important information link among all individuals directly involved with the patient.

Because of its logical, organized format, the POMR can facilitate self-audits and other patient care evaluation activities. The POMR is compatible with computer applications for medical records because of its standardized organization of information. Reluctance on the part of individuals to change their recording patterns may make it difficult to obtain acceptance of the POMR by the entire medical staff. One or more clinical services may elect to adopt or adapt to the POMR approach. The desirable features of the POMR should be considered when revising the current medical record structure. Implementing the POMR does require the support of the medical staff, support of administration for in-service training programs, and support of medical record practitioners, in converting from one method to another. Implementing the POMR must be carefully handled to prevent increases in costs and time spent because of documentation requirements.

Abbreviations

Abbreviations are commonly used in medical records. It is advisable that the hospital keep a record of those abbreviations it has approved for use. Clarity in the records is essential and cannot be obtained if some shorthand notes are comprehensible only to the author.

A list of symbols and abbreviations for use in medical records should be approved by the medical staff. Each abbreviation should have only one meaning. Diagnoses and procedures should be written in full, without the use of symbols or abbreviations. A legend should be included in the design of medical record forms when information recorded on the forms uses unique or a large number of abbreviations and symbols. Medical record practitioners should take the lead in ensuring that abbreviations are used in medical records only when appropriate and that abbreviations do not threaten the objective description of facts essential to both good medical practice and scientific progress.

Medical Record Content

Regardless of the method used in a hospital to record medical record information, the content of each medical record depends on which hospital department is treating the patient and recording information.

Inpatient Records

Neither JCAH nor AHA recommend any specific format or forms for use in hospital medical records. However, JCAH does establish requirements for medical record content to meet standards for sufficient information. Briefly, the requirements for inpatient records include:

- Patient identification data
- Medical history of patient, including chief complaint; present illness or injury; relevant past, family, and social histories; and inventory by body systems
- Report of relevant physical examination
- Diagnostic and therapeutic orders
- Clinical observations, including results of therapy as noted by physicians and others directly involved, consultations, and nurses' notes
- Reports of procedures, tests, and the results, including both diagnostic and therapeutic procedures
- Evidence of appropriate informed consent; when consent is not obtainable, the reason shall be entered in the record
- Conclusions at termination of hospitalization or evaluation or treatment, including any pertinent instructions for follow-up care

JCAH standards require the medical record to contain evidence of informed consent for procedures and treatment for which hospital policy requires informed consent. The policy on informed consent is developed by the medical staff and hospital governing board, consistent with legal requirements for an appropriate informed consent. The term *informed consent* is reserved for procedures and treatments. It implies that the patient has been informed of the procedure or operation to be done, of the risks involved, and of the possible consequences. By signing the consent, the patient or patient's representative indicates having been informed and consents to the procedure or treatment. An authorization for treatment, signed at the time of admission, is not to be confused with an informed consent. If, for some reason, the informed consent is not filed with the medical record, the medical record must indicate that an informed consent was obtained for a given procedure and treatment and the location of the informed consent.

Ambulatory Care Records

The record content requirements established by JCAH for hospital-sponsored ambulatory care services are:
- Patient identification data
- Relevant history of illness or injury and physical findings
- Diagnostic and therapeutic orders
- Clinical observations, including results of treatment
- Reports of procedures, tests, and the results
- Diagnostic impression or established diagnosis
- Patient disposition and any pertinent instructions given to the patient or family for follow-up care
- Immunization record
- Allergy history
- Growth charts for pediatric patients
- Referral information to and from outside agencies

- Any prior pertinent medical record information maintained by the hospital

The difficulties in maintaining standards for quality and content of ambulatory care records are often caused by the episodic nature of ambulatory care, the fragmentation of care that results from specialty clinics, and the rapid pace of outpatient care, which fosters brief entries of information. Innovations are needed in most hospitals to improve the ambulatory care information system.

Emergency Service Records

JCAH standards as well as legal considerations dictate that a medical record be maintained on every patient seeking emergency care and, where feasible, that the emergency record be incorporated into the patient permanent medical record. If the previous record is on microfilm or has been retired, incorporation is not possible. The medical record department must provide the services necessary to make previous inpatient, ambulatory care, and emergency service records available upon request of the attending physician or other persons authorized to request them.

Standards for information to be entered in the emergency service record include:
- Patient identification
- Time and means of arrival
- Pertinent history of illness or injury, physical findings, and vital signs
- Any emergency care given to the patient prior to arrival, such as that provided by the ambulance service
- Diagnostic and therapeutic orders
- Clinical observations, including results of treatment
- Reports of procedures and tests carried out
- Diagnostic impression
- Disposition of the patient, the patient's condition on discharge or transfer, and instructions given to the patient or family for follow-up care
- Medical advice given in the event the patient left against advice

Another record maintained in the emergency department is a control register, or log, for entering in chronological order by date and time the name of every individual seeking care. The individual's name is followed by age, sex, means of arrival, nature of complaint, disposition, and time of departure. Dead-on-arrival cases are also entered into the register. The register serves a number of purposes, such as for tabulation of statistical data on utilization of emergency services and types of cases and for selection of cases in assessing the quality of care.

Home Care Records

Standards for hospital-sponsored home care programs include the maintenance of accurate records for every patient receiving care through the program. The medical record requirements should be similar to those required for inpatients and ambulatory care patients. Professional staff members of the home care program must have access to the inpatient and ambulatory care records of their patients in the development of written patient care plans.

Information to be recorded in home care records includes:

- Designation of the physician having primary responsibility for the patient's care
- Composition of the patient's household and name of person who will assume responsibility when necessary
- Adequacy of the patient's residence for provision of required health care services
- Progress notes, signed and dated, for each home visit
- Copies of all transfer and summary reports
- Upon conclusion of home care services, a discharge report with disposition and any referral

In this particular type of record, the progress notes include documentation of signs and symptoms, treatment or service given, any medication administered, patient's reaction, any change in patient's condition, and any instructions given to the patient or family. A copy of the written summary report sent to the primary physician every 60 days is filed with the medical record.

Clarification of departmental areas of responsibilities for medical record services with the home health care program includes responsibility for record security and procedures for the orderly flow of medical records between inpatient, ambulatory care, and home health care facilities; for disclosure of medical record information to outside parties; for any recommended changes in forms design; and for dispatching records to and from home health care offices.

Skilled Care Facility Records

A hospital-administered skilled care facility may be located within the hospital or a distance from it, or a hospital may use the swing-bed method, which allows a hospital to change bed designation from acute care to skilled care and vice versa, depending on the level of care required by a patient.

With few exceptions, the same medical record forms can be used for both acute and skilled care. However, entries must be made on the front sheet of the record and in the body of the record to clearly identify the date of transfer to and from acute care and skilled care levels. For statistical and financial audit purposes, the medical record must differentiate between the two levels of care being provided. When the patient is transferred from the acute care level to the skilled care level, a summary of the acute care stay should be written. The instructions and orders for skilled care should be entered in the medical record.

If the skilled care facility is located a distance from the hospital, it may not be feasible to transfer a patient's entire medical record when the patient is transferred from acute care to skilled care. In this case, a clinical resume is prepared along with nursing care instructions and copies of any pertinent portions of the medical record for inclusion in the skilled nursing care facility's medical record.

For more information on standards for medical record services in long-term-care facilities, consult the latest edition of JCAH's *Accreditation Manual for Long-Term Care Facilities*.

Health Maintenance Organization Records

A hospital may have contractual arrangements with a health maintenance organization (HMO) to provide inpatient, emergency, and diagnostic services as requested and authorized by the HMO. Persons enrolled in an HMO are provided ambulatory care services, including preventive medicine, and inpatient care services as stipulated by the HMO plan.

Responsibility for the following areas must be clarified between the HMO and the hospital providing medical record services: procedures for the exchange of pertinent medical information, which is necessary for acute and continuing patient care, and procedures for the disclosure of medical record information to the patient or an outside party.

Hospice Records

Hospice care for terminally ill patients is an alternative to care in an acute care institution. The record system must be compatible with the care of terminally ill patients and the needs of the hospice. Medical record practitioners must be familiar with hospice services that are covered and reimbursable under Medicare, Medicaid, Social Services, and the Older Americans Act programs, as well as state licensing and health planning requirements.

Additional Department Patient Records

Evaluation and treatment records may be needed in a specific department to permit continuity of therapy or for departmental case studies and reports. While the patient is in the hospital, the daily records of physical therapy, occupational therapy, or social services may more easily be maintained in those departments, provided timely progress notes are entered in the patient's chart. The evaluation and treatment information should be incorporated in the patient's medical record when treatment or therapy has been completed, either by a summary or by inserting the actual documents. The department may wish to keep a copy of the information submitted to the patient medical record; however, the original document should be placed in the patient's permanent medical record.

Departmental work sheets designed for temporary use may be destroyed after pertinent information has been transferred to the patient's medical record. Work sheets containing notes that could be misinterpreted at a later date do not belong in the patient's medical record.

Chapter 5

Medical Record Forms

Medical record practitioners are responsible for assisting in the design and implementation of effective forms for data collection and use. Well-designed medical record forms are important communication tools and ready references in patient care and in review of care provided.

Forms should be designed to facilitate data collection as well as to provide complete and accurate data. Because of the costs of storage space and microfilming, as well as the difficulty of finding desired information in many records, it is imperative that good organization, conservation of paper, and effective methods of record indexing be carefully considered when selecting forms.

Neither the AHA nor JCAH recommends any specific medical record forms. Each hospital adopts the forms that best meet its needs. Medical record practitioners must work with other knowledgeable persons to develop forms that will promote adherence to standards for documenting patient care, will organize information for easy reference, will reduce wasted space, and will allow consideration of the individual hospital's needs.

In some communities, hospitals have worked together, through a representative committee, to adopt basic forms acceptable to their medical and hospital staffs and have thus made possible the economy of shared printing in quantity. Where physicians practice in more than one hospital, the use of the same record forms in all of the community's hospitals simplifies the recording procedure and promotes adherence to high standards. A cooperative spirit among medical record practitioners can assist in the development of common forms and result in improved documentation.

Medical record forms should be designed for use by those who are directly involved in patient care. Forms should be comprehensible to the staff members responsible for completing them and to the staff members who are guided by the recorded information in rendering patient care. Unnecessary duplication of entries in the record should be eliminated. For example, if the physician is required to list all diagnoses in the discharge summary, the face sheet could be designed to contain only admission information, patient identification data, and authorizations. The goal is to eliminate unnecessary pencil pushing, such as repetitive listing of some data, and to provide a succinct record that reflects high-quality care rendered.

Forms Committee

Because the authority to enter information in medical records is granted by the medical staff, medical record forms should be approved by a representative group of the medical staff, usually the medical record committee. The medical record committee may be the forms committee, or a hospital forms committee may be appointed to maintain an effective forms design and control program. The duties and authority of a forms committee should be clearly defined and supported by hospital administration. The medical record director may serve as chairman of the forms committee to coordinate all the tasks involved.

The committee should review forms, recommend changes in content, make changes in design to conform to an established basic record format (for example, standard location and sequence of identifying information and standard margins), and eliminate forms for which there is no need. If forms review is handled by the administrative forms committee, the medical record forms committee should coordinate its efforts with the other committee's.

A forms numbering system is necessary for easy identification and stock control. Samples of all editions of approved forms should be kept on file, and each form should be accompanied by a brief statement of its purpose and principal uses. The form number, the approval date, and the number ordered should be printed on each revision to ensure identification. A list of these assigned numbers, their titles, and the dates of approval for each of the forms is recommended; this list can also serve as a catalog. If there is a hospitalwide forms numbering system, the medical record forms numbering system should be coordinated with it.

In the development of a new form, it is advisable to have only a small supply of forms prepared for trial use, because experience frequently indicates a need for revisions. Since cost is also a factor in continually revising and printing small quantities of forms, photocopying or mimeographing might be the reproduction method of choice, depending on the number of copies needed. Forms should be kept simple and the variety few in number, to provide flexibility and reduce record bulk. All discontinued forms should be removed from the stockroom or supply area and destroyed.

Before developing a new form or revising an existing form, the steps shown in figures 1 and 2, pages 43 and 44, can be used to compile the necessary facts and to determine what, if any improvements should be made.

Principles of Forms Design

The following principles are basic to good forms design:

1. A uniform size of paper should be used. Although standard size 8½-inch by 11-inch paper is most commonly used, 8½-inch by 5½-inch paper could prove less wasteful.
2. A uniform binding edge should be maintained, either as a top or a side binding.
3. A uniform margin that is based on the binding edge should be maintained. Chart holders on the nursing units should accommodate the uniform margins.
4. For top binding, information on forms that are to be printed on both sides should be correctly placed on both sides for proper assembly in the chart. For side binding the two sides should be head-to-head.
5. Depending on whether the forms are to be typewritten, handwritten, or both, line spaces on forms should be assigned.
6. The quality and weight of paper should be selected according to the expected life of the record, the amount of use it will receive, and whether both sides are to be used. If both sides will be printed, the paper must be heavy enough to prevent the ink from showing through. A 20-pound stock is recommended for long-term use.
7. Colored forms should be selected carefully because problems can occur in photocopying or microfilming colored sheets. White paper with color-coded borders will prove more effective for quick identification of different forms in the hard-copy record.
8. Where feasible, the use of a rubber stamp on an existing form can be used to eliminate the need for a special form that is not used regularly.

Principles of Forms Development

The following principles are basic to good forms development:

1. There should be a demonstrated need and purpose for every item on the form. Items that "might be nice to have" or "may be needed some day" require collection time that is disproportionate to the value of the information.
2. Items should be listed in logical sequence. For example, it is logical to place age immediately following date of birth, and telephone number following address.

3. The horizontal space allowed for typewritten entries should accommodate the type size (pica or elite).

4. Spacing should be planned according to the method of documentation, whether it is typewritten, handwritten, or computer printout.

5. All forms should have the identification of the patient in a standard location.

6. When uniform placement is not feasible, there should be a uniform sequence of common items on related forms.

7. Terminology in item headings should be consistent on all forms.

8. Forms that require recopying or information from other parts of the record should be avoided.

9. The name of the hospital should be preprinted on all forms to identify any authorized photocopies used outside the hospital. To save space the name can be placed longitudinally in the left-hand margin of the form.

10. In certain areas of the form, the use of bold print for emphasis can be considered.

11. For easy identification, a form number should be printed on each form.

12. Forms should be designed to provide instructions on completion, which are placed on the top whenever possible (small print may be used). Routing instructions may be placed at the bottom. Use of symbols or abbreviations (as allowed) should have a legend, usually in the upper left corner.

13. Answer boxes can save time in completing the data for a form and can reduce errors as well as provide uniformity of statistical items. However, the item must be explicit to provide a meaningful "check-off" or "fill-in" box.

14. Prefabricated forms, such as "snap-out" or "multipart" forms should be considered whenever it is determined that a number of functions can be served by a single entry. Weigh the additional cost of the form against the saving of personnel time now required to handle one or more existing forms.

Carbon Copies

Carbon copies can be made, by hand or by typewriter, by inserting loose carbon sheets between forms or by using form pads with carbons already inserted. Snap-out forms can be used with a one-time carbon. This facilitates varying the contents of various parts of the form. Snap-out forms may cost more than the inserted carbons, but are faster to use and produce perfect alignment of written or typed matter on all copies. Forms with carbon backs are more expensive than forms with loose carbons, especially if the carbon is used only on portions of the form.

Figure 1. Gathering the Facts for Designing a New Form

Need

What procedures are accomplished by completion of this form? Does its use justify its existence?

On what other forms is this information duplicated in part or whole?

What inadequacies are there in completing this form or in performing the procedures?

Staff—Hospital and Medical

Who requires or needs this information in part or whole? Medical staff, individual physicians, other professional staff, patient accounts, administration, outside agencies, reimbursers?

Who enters the information?

Who will use this information? Will it be used in original, abstracted, or statistical form?

Location

Where is the form initiated, completed, and processed?

Where is the form sent and what is the distribution?

Where is the form filed?

Time

When is the information entered on the form?

What causes delays in completing the form?

Should the form be held in the unit pending completion?

When are the forms filed?

Method

How are data entered on the form—written, typed, word processing, microprocessor, or mainframe computer generated?

How is the information on this form distributed to other units needing the information in part or whole?

How many units are maintaining files for part or all of the information on this form? How many duplicate files are in departments of the hospital?

Figure 2. Improving an Existing Form

Need

Is the proposed information needed?

Does the cost of gathering or recording the information exceed its worth?

Is there a more reliable source or an easier way to obtain the information?

Can existing forms or the items on the form at hand be combined, eliminated, simplified, rearranged for better sequencing, or enlarged for additional items?

Staff—Hospital and Medical

Can the work of completing part or all of the form's data items be delegated to nonprofessional staff?

Can the handling or processing of the form be handled by other units or clerks to simplify the work? Can it be combined with other procedures for handling?

Can the data items be resequenced or revised to simplify entering and recalling or abstracting the data?

Location

Can the completion and processing of the form be better done in another unit or combined with similar work in another unit?

Can the form be designed to eliminate the need to initiate another form or having to make copies of the completed form, or copy forms on another form?

Can the form be better designed to assist in filing, retrieval, storage, and retirement (disposal)?

Time

Is there a more timely method for entering the information?

Can peak loads be leveled off by better scheduling of procedures to complete and process information?

Can a clerk be assigned to initiate the form by requesting information when it is available and process the procedure during slack times?

Method

Can the writing method be changed for ease and timeliness in completion?

Can the routing method be improved?

Has the form been developed to use the most efficient office equipment and to provide for an integrated information system now or in the future?

Can the information in this form be centralized for access by authorized persons, thus eliminating duplication of files?

No-carbon-required (NCR) forms are chemically treated papers that permit reproduction of typewritten or handwritten entries on one or more copies in a set of forms without the use of carbon paper. Their use may be preferable for certain applications. Because NCR sheets retain their reproducible characteristics, they should not be placed between other forms still in use in the medical record.

Continuous Forms

Continuous forms are often used by word processing units for transcribing histories and physical examinations, discharge summaries, and other dictation. The transcriptionist can type on continuous forms without stopping to remove and insert forms with carbons for each document transcribed. The forms can be separated and attached to the proper record at the end of the workday.

Reproduction Systems

Reproduction machines using master copies or stencils can produce more copies of forms and cards than is possible with carbon paper. This method will prove economical if the need arises for many copies. Care should be taken to avoid reproduction methods that result in poor-quality copies, especially if the form is to be used in the medical record.

A clinical service or a physician may request the hospital to prepare quantities of physician order sheets with printed standing orders, leaving blank the space for dosages of any listed medications. The physician will either enter the dosages or call them in and will sign the standing order. Such requests are made in the interest of starting patient care immediately after the patient's admission. Requests for printed standing order forms must have the approval of the medical record committee or other appropriate medical staff committee before the standing orders are printed.

Most hospitals have photocopying machines. Depending on the size and features, photocopying machines may be rented, rented with option to buy, or purchased. For most tasks that require more than one copy, photocopying requires less time than preparing carbon copies on a typewriter. Depending on the hospital size and the uses made of the copying machines, one or more machines should be located in the hospital for convenient use by medical record department staff. It is not unusual for the medical record department itself to have a photocopying machine. In terms of costs and advance planning required, the use of commercial photostating companies has limited value.

When copies of parts or all of a patient's medical record are sent to parties outside of the hospital, a rubber-stamped label or a permanent label should be affixed to one or more sheets stating "Any disclosure of medical record information by the recipient(s) is prohibited except when implicit in the purposes of this disclosure." No more patient information should be copied than is necessary to carry out the purpose of the disclosure.

Chapter 6

Review of the Medical Record

A patient's medical record is a compilation of various general and specialized medical record forms that contain information specific to the care of that patient. Timely reviews are conducted to determine completeness, accuracy, and adequacy of the information contained on these forms, using established standards as criteria. Two types of review are conducted: quantitative and qualitative analyses of documentation.

The quantitative and qualitative review of the medical record itself must be differentiated from activity directed at assessing the quality of medical care provided. In assessing the medical record for adequacy of documentation, medical record personnel must be careful to refrain from including judgments or assessments of the quality of care provided. The quantitative and qualitative review of the medical record will provide indications of the record's strengths and weaknesses for use in assessing the quality of medical care provided.

Quantitative Review

Quantitative review is conducted to determine the completeness of a medical record. It is a fact-gathering task to determine the presence or absence of data items, such as:

- Authentication (signatures) for all entries in the medical record (progress notes, physician orders, operative reports, and so forth)
- Operative report, anesthesia report, pathology report, and recovery room notes for patients requiring surgery
- Discharge summary
- History and physical examination report
- Reports of all diagnostic tests or studies ordered (laboratory, x-ray, EEG, EKG, and so forth)
- Prenatal report filed in obstetrical records

Check-off lists are developed for use by medical record personnel responsible for assembling the records of discharged patients and inspecting the records for absence of any required items. Deficiencies are noted on the check-off list and the medical record is routed to the appropriate staff member for completion. It is the department head's responsibility to maintain a current list of incomplete medical records by name of staff member responsible for completing the record. This list should also note the type of deficiency in each record. A monthly report should be submitted to the responsible physician, the medical record committee, the chief of the medical staff, and the hospital administrator that identifies the responsible physician, the medical records by record number, the types of deficiencies, and the length of time the records have remained incomplete. Each incomplete medical record should have a deficiency slip attached to the folder that indicates the deficiencies and the staff physician or person responsible for rectifying the deficiency. When the record is found to be complete, the deficiency slip is removed.

In some hospitals, the director of medical records has introduced a new approach in the maintenance of records to meet quantitative and qualitative standards. Medical record personnel with technical training or experience have been assigned to carry out quantitative and qualitative reviews of patient records on the nursing units. Daily or weekly checks are made to ascertain deficiencies and to notify responsible staff members of any existing deficiencies. In some instances, medical record personnel are provided with desks and necessary equipment on the nursing floors to transcribe physician reports, notes, and summaries. When this approach is used, the medical record may be assembled in permanent filing order, completed, abstracted, and coded within a few hours of the patient's discharge and then dispatched to the medical record department for further processing.

Quantitative reviews that find missing or late diagnostic reports necessitate further investigation by the department head to determine the reason. Delays in dispatching reports or problems on the nursing unit in getting the reports into patient medical records are cause for concern. To overcome these problems, it may be necessary for the director of medical records to assume the responsibility for supervising routine pickups, delivery, and placement of diagnostic reports in the patient charges on nursing units. This would be an added function for the department and may require more personnel but may not require as many personnel hours as are currently expended in tracking down missing reports.

Qualitative Review

The qualitative review of the medical record is often the by-product of quality assurance activities in assessing patient care. Medical record practitioners assisting the medical staff in abstracting the medical record for compliance with quality-of-care criteria often find the information is inadequate for abstracting. This should prompt the development of a fact-gathering list of inadequacies in the hospital medical records for purposes of quality assurance studies. The medical record committee or the quality assurance committee would use the data on inadequacies in activities to promote better documentation in the medical record.

Another approach to qualitative review is to develop significant points to be reviewed for qualitative documentation. Such a list can be developed by the medical record practitioner in cooperation with the medical record committee or a representative group of the medical staff and other professional staff. The results of such activity could indicate the need for better forms design, faster turnaround time in word processing, corrective action in documentation, and so forth.

Examples of questions to be asked in the qualitative review of the medical record are:

- Is the admitting office staff consistent and accurate in gathering data for entry on the front (face) sheet of the medical record?
- Does the history of present illness reflect the patient's words?
- Does the patient's history include references to any past history, family history, and review of systems as required in the criteria established for the qualitative review?
- Does the frequency of physician progress notes meet the criteria established for qualitative review?
- Do the physician progress notes describe the patient's problems, the patient's clinical state of comfort or distress, and reasons for therapeutic decisions?
- What is the time lapse between dictation and transcription of operative and other reports? Do these reports show dates of dictation and transcription?
- Do the nurses' notes meet the criteria established for quality review of documentation?
- Are the rules for making corrections of errors followed?
- Are rules for use of symbols and abbreviations followed?

Discharge Analysis

Discharge analysis is a term that designates the separate, daily tasks performed in processing for completion all of the medical records of patients discharged from the hospital. The words used to describe this activity vary from hospital to hospital. A brief description of the tasks involved follows.

Accounting for Records Due

A daily list of patients who have been discharged or who have died is prepared for internal distribution by the admitting office. Patients are listed by name, location, and medical record number. The medical record department receives one or more copies of the discharge list. It serves as a checklist in making sure that all records of discharged and dead patients have been received or are accounted for. Medical records of deceased patients may be in the pathology department if an autopsy has been performed. These records should be obtained as soon as possible. All records of previous admissions not returned with the current medical record must be obtained from the nursing units. If a card file is maintained for current inpatients, the cards of patients listed on the discharge list are pulled from the file.

Record Assembly

The requirements for documentation and access while the medical record is located in the nurses' station dictate a sequential order and arrangement for continuous updating and reference. When the medical records of discharged patients arrive in the medical record department, they are reassembled in an established order to provide a uniform format for ongoing use. The established order is that agreed upon by the medical staff (such as the medical record committee) in cooperation with the hospital's CEO. It is often referred to as the medical record format for permanent filing and includes any ambulatory care records on a patient within a single record. *Permanent* refers to the length of time medical records are to be maintained in their original or miniaturized form.

Arranging the medical record into component parts (medical, ancillary services, and nursing), with chronological filing within each component, is the source-oriented method for permanent format. Another method is to file all documentation in chronological order. This encourages users to read the entire record instead of spot-checking. The format of the medical record should promote ease in referencing needed information.

Labels placed on the folder of the medical record are used to immediately notify physicians and nurses about cautionary steps. Examples of such labels are "Allergy to Penicillin," "Anticoagulant Therapy," "Steroids," "Glaucoma Care," and so forth. The medical staff decides what labels may be used and who is responsible for placing them on the folders. The decision is usually based on the need to flag certain types of cases for precautionary measures in emergency services and ambulatory care clinics.

Record Completion

Procedures should be written for use in reviewing the medical record for completeness. A checklist can be developed for use in identifying those deficiencies that need physician entries. Another checklist can be developed to identify any commonly occurring deficiencies that need to be addressed by diagnostic, therapeutic, or nursing services. The purpose of the review is to promote a complete, accurate, and timely medical record. Highlights of the review process are presented below for use in developing procedures.

Admission Record. Information contained in the patient identification section of the front sheet varies in amount and specificity from hospital to hospital. Basic data to accurately identify a patient include name, residence, medical record number, age, date of birth, sex, race, marital status, name of nearest kin with address and telephone number, and religious preference. Also included on the front sheet prepared by the admitting office are admission date, room location or nursing unit assignment, source of payment, attending physician's name, type of admission, and admitting diagnosis or problem. The medical record department will enter the discharge date and any transfer of clinical service or physician. For emergency admissions, the admitting officers may not always have access to all patient identification information. Missing information is to be filled in as it becomes available.

All pages in the medical record should identify the patient by name, medical record number, and nursing unit or room number.

Discharge Summary or Note. The discharge summary is a concise recapitulation of the reasons for hospitalization, significant findings, procedures performed, course of hospitalization, condition of patient on discharge, and instructions given to the patient or family relating to physical activity, medications, diet, and follow-up care. A copy of diet instructions given to the patient should be entered in the medical record or a sample of it should be maintained on file in the medical record department for reference as necessary. The discharge plan of the social service department should be in the medical record. The medical staff should establish guides for obstetrical and newborn records that require discharge summaries instead of discharge notes, which contain a few sentences rather than a detailed report.

All diagnoses affecting the hospital stay are to be recorded in full either on the discharge summary or on the discharge form. The same is true for surgical and pertinent diagnostic procedures. No abbreviations should be used in documenting diagnoses and surgical procedures.

History and Physical Examination. Chief complaint, history of present illness, relevant past illnesses with social and family history, and inventory of body systems make up the history. The physical examination should reflect a comprehensive current physical assessment of the patient. The history and physical examination should be signed by the examining physician. If a complete physical examination was performed in the physician's office within a week of admission to the hospital, a durable, legible, signed copy of this report can be used in the hospital record, provided any change in the patient's physical status has been added to the report. A durable, legible copy of the office prenatal record is acceptable for obstetrical records.

An interval history and physical examination report is acceptable if the patient has been readmitted within 30 days of discharge for the same or related condition. This interval note should reflect any subsequent changes. The previous medical record should be on the nursing unit for access as necessary.

Pathology and Clinical Laboratory Reports. Signed, dated originals of reports of examinations by the pathologist and tests performed by laboratory personnel are placed in the medical record. When tests are performed by outside laboratory services contracted for by the hospital, the name of the laboratory performing the test is to be identified on the report placed in the patient's medical record. Reports of clinical laboratory forms are slips placed in shingle fashion on a full-size sheet. Slips should not overlap the test results. The test findings should be readily visible.

The pathologist, in cooperation with the medical staff, decides the exceptions for submission of specimens removed at surgery to the pathology laboratory and for specimens that require only macroscopic descriptions. The medical record department should be aware of these exceptions. Most surgical pathology reports will have both macroscopic and microscopic descriptions with diagnosis accompanying the microscopic findings. When an autopsy is performed, the report of provisional anatomic diagnoses should be filed in the medical record within three days and the complete necropsy protocol should be received and filed in the medical record within 90 days.

Radiologic and Other Diagnostic Laboratory Reports. Signed, dated originals of radiologic and other diagnostic reports are filed in the medical record. Authentication is by the person interpreting the film, tracing, tomography, ultrasound, or other process. These reports should be completed and filed in the medical record within 24 to 48 hours of the date of procedure. Arrangements should be made for any preadmission procedure reports to accompany the admission record to the nursing unit.

Anesthesia Record. A preanesthesia evaluation is necessary unless local anesthesia is to be used. This evaluation includes information on the choice of anesthesia, the surgical or obstetrical procedure anticipated, the patient's previous drug history, past anesthetic problems, and any potential anesthetic problems.

The anesthesia record describes the preoperative medication; the type and amount of anesthetic; the duration of anesthesia and procedure; the medications given in the operating room; and the condition of the patient, including pulse, respiration, and blood pressure throughout surgery. The record is signed by the anesthesiologist or anesthetist. Any difficulties or complications arising during administration of the anesthetic are recorded on the anesthesia form. The anesthesiologist's or the anesthetist's postoperative evaluation is also to be recorded on the anesthesia form or in the progress notes. The postanesthesia recovery note must include date and time of follow-up visit(s).

Operative Report. The preoperative diagnosis is recorded in the record before sugery. Operative reports should be dictated immediately following surgery. The report includes the date of the operation, names of primary surgeon and any assistants, description of the findings, technical procedure carried out, tissue removed, condition of the patient at the completion of the procedure, and the postoperative diagnosis. When a house officer serves as assistant surgeon and dictates the operative report, the primary surgeon is responsible for authenticating the report.

The dictated operative report should be transcribed immediately and placed in the patient's record for reference by those directly involved in the patient's care. The dates of dictation and transcription should be recorded on the operative note. If there are delays in transcribing the operative reports, the surgeon should enter a brief description of the surgery in the progress note section.

Progress Notes. Signed, dated entries reflecting the course of the patient's illness or injury during hospitalization are the responsibility of the physician(s) and other staff members authorized to write progress notes. The frequency with which progress notes are written depends on the patient's condition and the medical staff's rules or guidelines for progress notes. Records of patients hospitalized for more than four hours that do not contain progress notes should be reviewed by the medical record committee. The medical record department has the responsibility of calling record deficiencies to the attention of the medical record or quality assurance committee.

Should the course of hospitalization be complicated, the progress notes need to identify the complications and indicate the procedures and tests initiated, the types of problems being evaluated and ruled out, and the patient's response to the treatment modes initiated. The physician's progress notes should indicate that the physician has read the nurses' notes.

Physicians' Orders and Nurses' Medication. Diagnostic and therapeutic orders are dated and signed by the responsible physician or dentist. The authority of physicians and dentists in training and other practitioners within the hospital to write diagnostic and therapeutic orders is in accordance with state licensure laws and clinical privileges granted by the organized medical staff. Medication orders of unlicensed house officers may require countersignatures by a medical staff member. Hospital and medical staff rules will identify those who are qualified to accept and transcribe verbal orders. The medical staff should have a written list of orders that require authentication by the responsible physician within 24 hours of a verbal order; these are medications and procedures that could be hazardous to the patient. A discharge order should be written before the patient's discharge from the hospital.

The medication chart may be incorporated with the doctors' order sheet or it may be a separate form. In some hospitals, the medication order form has multiple parts, with copies for the pharmacy and the physician. The original medication order and administration form is filed in the patient's medical record. Nurses record the time and date of medication administration and either initial or sign the entry. If the nursing service director permits the nurses to initial their entries, the nursing service must be able to identify the individual nurses by initials.

Nursing Records. Clinical nursing records consist of assessment, planning, intervention, and evaluation. Nursing staff entries in the medical record should reflect this process for each inpatient. The assessment of the patient's needs is done at the time of admission to the nursing unit and is the plan of care to be carried out by the nursing staff.

On the basis of this assessment, the nursing department sets goals for each patient. A plan of care must be documented, and it should reflect current standards of nursing practice. The plan includes physiological, psychosocial, and environmental factors; patient and family education; and patient discharge planning.

Nursing documentation in the medical record should be pertinent and concise, reflecting the patient's status. It should document the patient's needs, problems, capabilities, and limitations. When the patient is transferred to another nursing unit or is discharged from the hospital, a nurse should document the patient's status in the record. The record should also reflect any discharge instructions given to the patient or the patient's representative.

The hospital should establish a policy regarding the frequency and method of recording nursing reports. Nursing forms can be developed to streamline nursing documentation by having a check-off column for routine services rendered. Nurses' notes should be limited to meaningful observations. They may be recorded on a separate form or on an integrated all-purpose progress form. Generally, nurses' notes include graphic charting of vital signs, such as temperature, pulse, and respiration; blood pressure readings; intake and output reports as necessary; and medications and treatments given.

Nursing care plans may be kept separate from the patient medical record, for example, on 5-inch by 8-inch cards at the nursing unit. This information may or may not become a part of the record. If the necessary information is recorded elsewhere in the record, the cards may be retained temporarily as determined by hospital policy, and then destroyed. If information documented on the nursing care plan is not reflected in the record, the cards should become a part of the patient's permanent medical record.

Short Stays. A condensed medical record may be maintained for patients who require less than 48 hours of hospitalization. The record should contain patient identification data, a description of the patient's condition, pertinent physical findings, an account of the treatment given, and other data necessary to justify the diagnosis and treatment. A discharge summary is not required. The attending physician may request the services of another physician or a specialist for consultation in diagnosis or treatment. The consultant's services may consist of tests, evaluations, and recommendations for diagnosis or treatment.

A consultation is usually initiated by a written order or request from the attending physician to another physician or specialty department. The request states the purpose and the nature of the consultation desired and gives pertinent clinical information. The report of the consultant's findings, evaluations, and recommendations are usually recorded on a consultation or progress note form, but special forms are used for certain types of examinations and tests, such as psychological tests, muscle strength tests, tests of levels of function for activities of daily living, and food histories. The request for a consultation and the original report of the consultant are filed in the patient's chart. The consultant may request a copy of the report for reference purposes.

Social Service Reports. Social service reports may contain intimate details of the patient's personal life, some of which may be hearsay prejudicial to the patient or misinterpreted at a later date by others reading the report. Therefore, the hospital may prefer to have the social service department prepare an interpretive summary for the patient's record that contains only the information of value to the physician and other professional personnel who contribute to the patient's care. The sensitive information is then kept in the social service department.

The Society for Hospital Social Work Directors of the American Hospital Association has published a book entitled *Documentation by Social Workers in Medical Records.* The guide states on page 6 that "The social worker must distinguish carefully between those facts observed and reported and those that are interpretative and diagnostic entries. The content should provide the background, social information, and problems that the patient, his family, and the social worker identify. The social worker should indicate the plan he has developed and the action and progress that do or do not occur. There should be a discharge note and/or an outcome statement, as well as provision for follow-up reports as needed."

Sensitive Information. Psychiatric intake reports and personal or family social information that could be detrimental to the patient or the patient's family if circulated may be filed separately to provide a greater degree of confidentiality. However, the medical record should include a note indicating where this information is filed and who should be contacted for access to it when it becomes necessary. The advice provided to social workers on page 8 of *Documentation by Social Workers in Medical Records* relative to principles and ethical aspects of recording serves as a guide to all health care professionals: "The social worker's judgment about what to record must be exercised in accordance with the type of social work activity and the goal of medical care. The social worker usually has access to a wealth of information about the patient, not all of which needs to be recorded in detail. The worker must record sufficient information to document his plan and actions with the patient and provide the other members of the team with relevant information. Highly sensitive and confidential information that is not necessary for the work of the other members of the team should be recorded in general rather than specific."

Chapter 7

Indexes and Registers

Hospitals maintain various indexes and registers so that patient medical records and other information can be located and classified for patient care purposes, case studies, utilization management and other administrative purposes, and for compliance with state regulations or licensure requirements.

Master Patient Index

The master patient index (MPI) is a file that identifies patients and their medical records that are maintained by the hospital. All patients registered to receive hospital care as an inpatient, outpatient, emergency service patient, or home care patient are to be entered in individually identifiable form in the MPI. The MPI file may consist of paper cards (1½ inches by 3 inches or 3 inches by 5 inches) housed in filing cabinets, or the file may be kept on a computer-assisted or microfiche system. Regardless of the mechanism used for filing, the MPI should contain sufficient information to readily identify a patient and that patient's medical record number.

The minimum data set for patient identification in the MPI is:
- Last name, first name, and middle initial
- Birthdate by month, day, and year
- Sex
- Address by street, city, state, and zip code
- Date of admission or registration
- Name of attending physician or clinical service assignment
- Medical record number

More information may be added as needed, such as the Social Security number for Medicare beneficiaries. In automated systems where updating of information is relatively easy and not too time-consuming, the dates of admission and discharge as well as clinic and emergency service visits may be entered. When the MPI also serves as the core of a computer-assisted patient account and clinical data system, more data items may be entered to serve various needs. Entering and storing data, whether on paper or in a computerized system, is expensive; therefore, only information whose use has been justified should be kept. Provision should be made for cross-referencing name changes, such as changing a single to a married name, and correcting errors in a name or birthdate.

There is no recommended period for retention of names in the MPI. The preservation of patient names and identification items usually exceeds the retention period for hospital medical records and is often regarded as a permanent file.

The filing arrangement within the MPI may be one of two systems. In the first system, the patient names are filed in alphabetical order by last name with secondary alphabetical filing by first name, such as:

Johansen, Charles

Johanssen, Amy

Johanssen, Charles

Johnson, Arthur

Johnson, Charles

The second system, which is used by many hospitals that serve communities with a diversity of last names, is the phonetic filing arrangement. Phonetic filing is better known by its trade name, Soundex, a product that Remington-Rand Office Systems originated. The name Soundex is now used by many vendors of phonetic filing systems. The phonetic filing system is based on retaining the first letter of the last name for the first order of filing and then translating the next three types of consonants into a three-digit code based on following arrangement of similar sounding consonants:

Consonants	Type Assignment
b, f, p, v	1
c, g, j, k, q, s, z, x	2
d, t	3
l	4
m, n	5
r	6

In the phonetic system, a,e,i,o,u,w,h, and y are all treated as vowels. When consonants within the same type assignment appear in consecutive order, only one digit is assigned for that type of consonant. If a name contains one or two types of consonants, one or two 0s are added to produce three digits. Mary Jane Doe would be assigned D-000, Mary. Examples of the phonetic filing system follow.

Name	Code Assignment (First file order)	Secondary File Order
Agee, Deloris	A-200	Deloris
Aigew, Doris	A-200	Doris
Agew, Doris	A-200	Doris
Bissenger, Olga	B-252	Olga
Basengelman, Olga	B-252	Olga
Johanssen, Charles	J-525	Charles
Johnson, Charles	J-525	Charles
Janssen, Robert	J-525	Robert
Olsen, John	O-425	John
Olson, John	O-425	John
Orlee, Claude	O-640	Claude
Quackenbush, Jacob	Q-251	Jacob
Quandt, Rose	Q-530	Rose
Quant, Rose	Q-530	Rose
Sanchez, Jaimee	S-520	Jaimee
Sanchoz, James	S-520	James

Last name, first name, and birthdate usually suffice for ready identification of most patients when the phonetic filing system is used. Variations of the phonetic filing system have been developed for use in a computerized patients' index, pharmacy index or formulary of drugs, and other name-type indexes.

The responsibility for quality control of the MPI should be delegated to the manager of the medical record department, whether the index is maintained on a manual or on a computer-assisted system. Patient identification data items should be audited for correct spelling, completeness of required data items, and correctness of filing order. In a manual system, colored audit cards taller than the index cards are used to accompany the index cards during filing. The newly filed index cards are then checked for accuracy of filing and the audit card is removed. The MPI, whether a manual or computer-assisted system, must be monitored for accuracy and adherence to the minimum data requirements. Written procedures are needed for handling any duplication in medical record number assignments (two patients with the same number), issuance of a new unit number to a patient with previously assigned unit number, and corrections or updating of data items.

Personnel in both admitting and medical records must be made aware of the importance of accuracy and completeness of data obtained at the time of admission and entered into the MPI. The MPI is the key to retrieval of medical records for patient-care purposes. It also contains the demographic items that, once entered into a computerized system, provide the core data for use in patient account and case-mix statistical studies.

Disease and Operation Index

The disease and operation index is a list arranged by illness, injury, and procedure that gives the numbers of patients' medical records in which information on specific illnesses, injuries, or procedures may be found. It is a cross-reference by disease, injury, and significant procedures to hospital medical records. The index is a tool for locating medical records by subject matter to carry out activities related to the following:

- Continuing medical education programs
- Epidemiologic and biomedical studies
- Health services research studios
- Statistical data on occurrence rates, ages, sex, and complications or associated conditions
- Patient care evaluation and quality control measures
- Consultation on patient response to treatment in previous cases for applicability in current case
- Review of medical records for compliance with accreditation standards, licensing standards, and regulatory requirements for adequacy of documentation

The disease and operation index is accessible only to authorized personnel. Posting data to the index requires personnel trained in checking for accuracy in entering data from the source document. Control measures are needed to ensure that every inpatient medical record is accounted for in the disease and operation index. Since quality assurance activities now include outpatient department and emergency service patient care, provision must also be made for retrieving these outpatient and emergency records by diagnoses, either by a separate index or by merging with the existing index.

The number of data items to be included in the disease and operation index depends on the needs of the individual hospital. When the disease and operation index is a product of a multiple-purpose discharge abstract system, more data is available as needed through computer printout displays. Basic data for any type of disease and operation index include the disease, injury, and procedure classification code; the patient's medical record number; sex and age of patient; identification of responsible physician by code or name; dates of admission and discharge or year with length of stay in days; any outcome of death and any autopsy; and associated disease or procedure codes. If a manual index is maintained, the number of data items should be kept to the minimum needed for record retrieval purposes. Adding data not used requires use of costly personnel time.

A manual index may be maintained on lined 5-inch by 8-inch cards in a vertical or visible filing cabinet or on 8½-inch by 11-inch lined paper in a three-ring loose-leaf binder. The minimum data for each diagnosis is posted on the appropriate card or sheet labeled for that diagnosis. When a patient has more than one diagnosis, the diagnoses are cross-referenced. For example, if the diagnoses on a discharged patient's record were acute myocardial infarction and diabetes mellitus, each diagnosis would be posted on its card or sheet and each would show the other condition as an associated disease. If two or more procedures were performed, each procedure would be posted on its card with a listing of other procedures performed. Posting to the index should be done daily, if possible, but only after the attending or responsible physician has recorded the diagnoses determined at the conclusion of the hospital stay.

If a hospital-based, computer-assisted health data system exists, the disease and operation index should be a product of the system. Hospitals subscribing to a system's discharge abstract system receive disease and operation index printouts periodically. Medical record practitioners should be aware of the various systems and services available and, where possible, take advantage of the automated systems that offer services and flexibility in providing data for multiple-purpose use.

Physician Index

The physician index is a list arranged by physician names (codes that identify individual physicians) that gives the medical record numbers of patients who received treatment or consultation from a particular physician. The minimum data requirements for entry on each physician's list is the patient's medical record number, patient's age and sex, date of admission and length of stay in days, identification of patient death and any autopsy, and whether any surgical procedure was performed. Data items on consultation entries usually require only the patient's medical record number, date of admission, and identification of the entry as a consultation provided to another physician's patient.

The physician index is regarded as a confidential record, and access to it is limited to authorized persons. Physicians have the right of access to their own data recorded in the physician's index. The hospital governing board and chief executive officer have the right of access in accordance with their duties and responsibilities for ensuring quality of patient care and conduct of hospital affairs. The credentials committee of the organized medical staff has the right of access as it relates to staff reappointment and reappraisal of privilege delineation. Only the hospital CEO, usually in cooperation with the executive committee or chief of medical staff, can authorize access by other persons and disclosure of data in physician-identifiable form.

One recent use of data from the physician index is the tabulation of data in physician-coded form to determine patient admission and length-of-stay rates by individual physicians in hospital-conducted utilization management studies. The physician index also serves as the tool for retrieval of patient medical records by physician. These studies must be authorized by the hospital CEO.

The physician index may be maintained on a manual file, using a card file or a loose-leaf binder. The physician index can also be generated as a product of a hospital-based computerized health data system or a hospital subscription to a discharge abstract service. When the physician index is part of an automated discharge abstract system, a variety of statistical studies on utilization of hospital services can be carried out in less time and with greater ease than could be accomplished with a manual system.

Cancer Registry

The cancer registry requires maintaining an index of patient names and addresses for follow-up studies on the outcome of malignancy, a statistical index on the type and site of malignancy with cross-referencing to the patient's medical record, and a patient's record of history and treatment, when applicable. A hospital that has no formal cancer program need not maintain a cancer registry. The American College of Surgeons (ACS) grants approval of cancer programs in hospitals based on compliance with ACS guidelines. In some states, the cancer registry program is carried out at the state level and hospitals cooperate by submitting abstract data from patient medical records.

Other Special Indexes

Special subject indexes may be maintained by the hospital, but the need for these indexes should first be justified based on interest and actual use of the data. Hospitals with trauma or burn centers may wish to maintain an index that provides specific statistical data on treatment provided and on utilization of the specialized service.

An index or log may be maintained to identify the organs or tissues removed from brain-death patients for transplantation purposes. The index should identify the patient's medical record number, the organ(s) or tissue removed, date of the procedure, and identification of any outside team who performed the procedure. The procedure is referred to as "harvesting" organs or tissue when it will be transplanted in another patient. In hospitals where the transplantation procedures are performed, the medical record department may wish to cross-reference the recipient's medical record number on the donor's entry.

Special indexes can be established to meet the needs of individual or groups of staff physicians. These are often needed only temporarily and steps should be taken yearly to determine if the index is still needed and is being used.

Hospitals with family medicine or primary care programs have an interest in maintaining a statistical data system that involves an index of diagnoses with reference to patient medical record numbers. The data items collected relate to services provided, treatment, findings or diagnoses, and professional staff directly involved in providing the care and services. The *International Classification of Health Problems in Primary Care (ICHPPC)* provides a short list of problems and diagnoses for use in maintaining this type of index. In addition, a list, selected by the program director, of patients' reasons for encounter may be used.

Registers

The need to maintain certain types of registers or logs may be determined by the requirements for record control measures or by state regulations imposed on the hospital.

The patient register or admission register is a chronological list of patient names by date of admission as inpatients. Minimum data items required are date of admission, time of admission if needed, patient name, and medical record number. Additional items may include room assignment, sex, and attending physician's name. If the admitting or medical record department prepares a daily list of admissions and hospital births, a copy may be filed to serve as an admission register. In some states, the hospital licensing laws may include requirements for a patient registration log (admission register).

It is important to maintain a control register or log of medical record number assignments. This register is a chronological list of medical record numbers with the name of the patient to whom each number was assigned. This control measure ensures that two or more patients have not been assigned the same medical record number. Immediate steps must be taken to correct errors in medical record number assignments.

The operating room register is a chronological list of all operative procedures performed in the hospital's surgical suite. It is usually maintained in the operating room suite area and contains the date and time of the procedure, the name of the patient, the type of procedure performed, the type of anesthesia used, and the names of the surgeon and anesthesiologist. The operating room register may be required by state regulations; however, it serves the hospital as a valuable reference for certain types of statistical data on utilization of services and human resources.

A chronological list is maintained on all hospital births. This birth register may be kept in the delivery room or obstetrical area or in the medical record department. It may be simple or detailed, depending on the needs of the obstetrical service and the hospital. The minimum data would be date and time of birth, sex of newborn, whether baby was born live or stillborn, name of mother, name of physician or staff member in attendance at the time of delivery, and date when birth certificate was mailed to the registrar of vital records. A birth register may be required by state vital record law.

A death register may be maintained in the medical record department, pathology department, or admitting office. It is a chronological list of all patients who died in the hospital or who were dead on arrival at the hospital. It contains the date of death, name of the deceased person, name of physician who completed the medical portion of the death certificate, and the name of the mortician, coroner, or medical examiner who removed the body from the hospital. The mortician has the responsibility for completing the remainder of the death certificate and for filing it with the registrar of vital records. When the body is removed by the coroner or medical examiner for examination, the medical portion of the death certificate is completed by the examiner. The hospital obtains a receipt for the body from the party who removes the deceased patient and this receipt may be filed in either the deceased patient's medical record or in the pathology department file.

A register is maintained in the emergency department to record patient encounters by date. The minimum data items to be entered in the emergency service register are the date and time of arrival, name of patient, means of transportation to the emergency service, treatment or advice given, disposition, and time of departure. The emergency department register does not preclude the need of an emergency service record on every patient treated. An entry in the emergency department register is needed on all dead-on-arrival cases, but an emergency service record is not opened when medical care is not given. Statistical data can be compiled monthly from the emergency department register to gauge utilization of emergency services.

Hospitals with computerized programs for processing admitting, discharge, and health care data should be able to produce most of these registers or logs. When registers or logs can be handled as a part or product of a health data system, manual registers should be eliminated.

Chapter 8

Diagnostic and Procedural Classification Systems

Diagnostic and procedural data can be classified in many ways, depending on the purpose of the classification system and the use being made of it. The most efficient classification system for hospitals is one that yields adequate information about large numbers of inpatients and ambulatory care patients and permits retrieval of the maximum number of patient medical records with review of the minimum number of records. A perfect design for classifying diagnoses, surgical procedures, and pertinent nonsurgical procedures would anticipate every request for health data information and patient record retrieval in all hospitals that use it. Such a system has not been designed and may be impossible to attain.

Classification systems presently used in the health care field range from those statistical in nature to those that are a catalog of terms for describing and recording clinical, pathological, or procedural terms. Although one classification system predominates in hospitals, medical record practitioners should be familiar with the existence and purpose of other classification and listing systems designed for use in the health care field.

International Classification of Diseases

The *International Classification of Diseases (ICD)* is a publication of the World Health Organization. Revisions are scheduled every ten years, and the ninth revision (*ICD-9*) is currently in use. Starting with the seventh revision of *ICD*, adaptations or modifications of *ICD* have been made in the United States for use in hospitals. The *International Classification of Diseases, Ninth Revision, Clinical Modification (ICD-9-CM)* is used in hospitals and *ICD-9* is used in state and federal agencies responsible for preparing vital statistics on births, deaths, and fetal deaths.

ICD-9-CM is a statistical classification designed to furnish quantitative diagnostic and procedural data on groups of cases. It is not a nomenclature, which allows for specificity in describing all approved clinical and pathological terminology. Medical record personnel must work with a variety of diagnostic and operative terminology used within one hospital that may be traced to the terminology patterns of various medical schools or clinical specialties and to the span of ages among physicians. ICD-9 and ICD-9-CM provide for all terms, good and bad, in classifying information from vital records and hospital medical records.

ICD-9-CM represents a series of necessary compromises among classifications based on etiology, anatomical site, age, and circumstances of onset. It was developed to provide a statistical compilation of illnesses and injuries. In addition, it provides a supplemental classification for factors influencing health status and contact with health services, a supplemental classification for classification of external causes of injuries, and a classification of surgical and nonsurgical procedures. Diseases are grouped according to the problems they present, with specific disease entities given separate titles or code numbers only when their separation is warranted because frequency of occurrence or importance as a morbid condition justifies assigning a separate category. Conditions of lower frequency or less importance are grouped together, often as residual groups of a particular anatomical site or physiological system. This arrangement results in a relatively simple numerical code and a statistical classification that serves the major needs of hospitals.

The Joint Commission on Accreditation of Hospitals recommends use of ICD or a modification thereof for indexing hospital medical records by diagnoses and operations. The Health Care Financing Administration (HCFA) requires the use of ICD-9-CM by hospitals in reporting diagnostic and procedural data for payment of services given to Medicare recipients. State Medicaid agencies also require hospitals to use ICD-9-CM in reporting data for reimbursement purposes. More and more insurance carriers are turning to ICD-9-CM for use in hospital reporting.

ICD-9-CM is published in three volumes, the Tabular List, Alphabetic Index, and Procedure Classification, and can be ordered from the U.S. Government Printing Office. The American Hospital Association maintains a central office on ICD-9-CM in cooperation with the United States Public Health Service National Center for Health Statistics and the American Medical Record Association to answer coding questions and to promote the use of ICD-9-CM among hospitals. The American Hospital Association publishes educational materials for use by hospitals in training personnel to code with ICD-9-CM, such as the ICD-9-CM Coding Handbook for Entry-Level Coders.

International Classification of Diseases for Oncology

International Classification of Diseases for Oncology (ICD-O) is a publication of the World Health Organization that provides for coding both the topography and morphology (histology) of tumors. *ICD-9-CM* contains, in chapter 2, a principally topographic code for neoplasms with an arrangement to identify the behavior (malignant, benign, in situ, and so forth). Only a few tumors are identified by histologic type in *ICD-9-CM*.

There is a close relationship between *ICD-O* and *ICD-9*, since the topography section of *ICD-O* is based on the malignant neoplasm categories 140-149 in *ICD-9*. A conversion table between *ICD-O* and *ICD-9* has been prepared by the National Cancer Institute of the National Institutes of Health (NIH publication No. 79-2007). *ICD-O*'s morphology section includes many code numbers for different histologic types of neoplasms and their synonyms.

ICD-O is used in cancer registry programs and in other programs requiring more specificity than is provided in *ICD-9-CM*. *ICD-O* may be ordered from the World Health Organization Publications Center for the USA, 49 Sheridan Ave., Albany, New York 12210.

Diagnostic and Statistical Manual of Mental Disorders

The *Diagnostic and Statistical Manual of Mental Disorders, Third Edition (DSM-III)*, is published by the American Psychiatric Association. *DSM-III* features diagnostic criteria, a multiaxial approach to evaluation of mental disorders, expanded descriptions of disorders, additional categories not included in *ICD-9*, and elimination of some categories contained in *ICD-9*. It is a statistical classification and glossary with more specificity than is contained in *ICD-9*, and it purports to reflect the most current knowledge regarding mental disorders. It is not completely compatible with *ICD-9-CM*, although the original intent of the *DSM-III* task force was to maintain compatibility.

DSM-III is used in many psychiatric institutions and psychiatric units of hospitals for indexing records by mental disorders and for compiling statistical data on patient care. Since *ICD-9-CM* is required for use in Medicare and Medicaid reimbursement reporting, medical record practitioners in psychiatric institutions and hospitals with psychiatric units need working knowledge of both *ICD-9-CM* and *DSM-III*.

International Classification of Health Problems in Primary Care

The *International Classification of Health Problems in Primary Care, 2nd edition (ICHPPC-2)*, is an adaptation of *ICD-9* intended for use in general medicine. It was prepared by the classification committee of the World Organization of National Colleges, Academies, and Academic Association of General Practitioners / Family Physicians in collaboration with the World

Health Organization. *ICHPPC-2* is published by the Oxford University Press and is available from its New York division.

ICHPPC-2 is designed to group the problems that make up primary medical care. It can be used to provide reliable statistical comparisons between morbidity or patient workloads of primary care physicians in the United States and around the world. *ICHPPC-2* contains 300 categories of health problems, has an optional hierarchy principle to accommodate the classification of problems of local importance and of special interest, has a full spectrum of first contact with health care providers ranging from rural practice to hospital emergency departments, contains the brevity and simplicity needed for use by coding personnel, and is closely aligned with *ICD-9-CM*. Perfect conversion of *ICHPPC-2* to *ICD-9-CM* is not possible. *ICHPPC-2* is used in the family medicine programs of many hospitals.

International Classification of Impairments, Disabilities, and Handicaps

The *International Classification of Impairments, Disabilities, and Handicaps* is a publication of the World Health Organization that was published in 1980 for trial purposes. It is a manual of classification relating to the consequences of diseases. The manual contains three distinct and independent classifications, each relating to a different plane of experience that is a consequence of a disease or injury. Impairments (I-code) are concerned with abnormalities of body structure and appearance and with organ or system function resulting from any cause (representing disturbances at the organ level). Disabilities (D-code) reflect the consequences of impairment in terms of functional performance and activity by the individual. Handicaps (H-code) are concerned with the disadvantages experienced by the individual as a result of impairments and disabilities (the ability to interact or adapt to surroundings).

Rehabilitation services are interested in using a manual such as this and have a strong need for classification to supplement diagnostic categories in *ICD-9-CM*. However, the manual has not been approved for use in official reporting to government agencies and reimbursement systems. It is a trial manual, subject to many changes before it becomes final.

Systematized Nomenclature of Medicine

Systematized Nomenclature of Medicine (SNOMed), second edition, is a publication of the College of American Pathologists. It is a nomenclature that catalogs approved terms for describing and recording clinical and pathological observations. It is extensive, so that any pathological condition can be accurately recorded, and it is capable of being expanded to include new terms necessary to record new observations. Any morbid condition that can be specifically described has a specific designation, using fields of information. In *SNOMed*, terms with numerical assignments are

68

cataloged by topography, morphology, etiology, function, disease, procedures, and occupations. The complete specificity of a nomenclature prevents *SNOMed* from serving satisfactorily as a statistical classification. A statistical classification of disease must be confined to a limited number of categories that will encompass the entire range of morbid conditions. *SNOMed* and its parent classification system, *Systematized Nomenclature of Pathology (SNOP)* are used in part or whole by many pathologists.

Current Procedural Terminology

Physicians' *Current Procedural Terminology (CPT)* is a publication of the American Medical Association. *CPT* is a listing of descriptive terms and identifying codes for reporting medical services and procedures performed by physicians. The purpose of *CPT* is to provide uniform terminology to accurately designate medical, surgical, and diagnostic services for communication among physicians, patients, and third parties. It is used in payment systems for services provided by physicians. Each service and procedure is identified with a five-digit code. There are sections for medicine, anesthesiology, surgery, radiology, and pathology and laboratory. Using *CPT*, the physician can report in coded form the place and type of physician-patient encounter, the diagnostic procedures performed, and the surgical procedure performed. By arrangement with the American Medical Association, the Health Care Financing Administration is expanding the sections in *CPT* to include services and procedures provided by other health care professionals entitled to reimbursement for services rendered to Medicare recipients. *CPT* provides greater detail for many procedures than hospitals need and for other procedures, provides less specificity than hospitals need. The alphabetical index of *CPT* does not lend itself to easy use by hospital coders.

Current Medical Information and Terminology

Current Medical Information and Terminology (CMIT) is a publication of the American Medical Association. It serves as a reference in identifying, describing, recording, and reporting disease entities and their diagnoses in programs for computerization of medical information. It is now in its fifth edition. The latest edition of *CMIT* may serve as a valuable reference in the medical record department, along with medical dictionaries used by coders and transcriptionists.

Standard Nomenclature of Athletic Injuries

The *Standard Nomenclature of Athletic Injuries* is a publication of the American Medical Association. This is another publication that can serve as a valuable reference for use by coders and transcriptionists in hospitals.

Symptom Classification

The Division of Health Resources Utilization Statistics of the National Center for Health Statistics developed *Symptom Classification* for use in the National Ambulatory Medical Care Survey (DHEW publication No. (HRA) 74-1337, Vital and Health Statistics Series 2, No. 63). The purpose was to classify patients' reasons for seeking health care. The World Health Organization is working on a classification of patients' reasons for seeking ambulatory medical care. For further information on this classification system, write to the Center for ICD in North America, National Center for Health Statistics, 3700 East-West Highway, Hyattsville, MD 20782.

Chapter 9

Quality Assurance

Professional Standard Review Organizations (PSROs) were established in 1972 by the Department of Health, Education, and Welfare (now the Department of Health and Human Services) to ensure peer review in evaluating necessity, quality, and cost-effectiveness of health care financed through federal programs. Even long before this, the term *quality assurance* was part of the vocabulary of every medical record practitioner.

The term PSRO is now outdated. The Tax Equity and Fiscal Responsibility Act of 1982 in section 1153(a)(i) created "utilization and quality control peer review organizations," or PROs. The act mandates the Secretary of Health and Human Services to designate geographic areas, generally so that each state is one area except in locations where there are at least 60,000 total hospital admissions annually. Hospitals must contract with a PRO in their area on or after October 1, 1984. The functions to be conducted by PROs are similar to the functions of the PSROs, including reviewing professional activities with regard to provision of services and determining whether payment should be made.

The Joint Commission on Accreditation of Hospitals (JCAH) has been involved in formal quality assurance from the first medical audits through establishment of its current quality assurance standards. JCAH standards require that hospitals have a quality assurance program and that they demonstrate an ongoing effort to deliver the best patient care possible with the available resources and consistent with achievable goals. The current JCAH quality assurance standards emphasize that:

- Hospitals must have a formal quality assurance program
- This program must be reflected in a written quality assurance plan
- The plan must contain mechanisms to evaluate patient care
- A comprehensive, hospitalwide quality assurance program is valuable

71

- Approaches to problem identification, assessment, and resolution should be flexible
- Focusing quality assurance activity on problems in areas in which the solutions have a potentially significant impact on patient care is important
- Focusing quality assurance activity on areas in which demonstrable problem resolution is possible is important
- The quality assurance program be coordinated by a committee, an individual, or a department

The JCAH standards also encourage the use of multiple data sources to identify problems and discourage the use of quality assurance studies for the sole purpose of documenting high-quality care.

Medical record practitioners should work with the hospital and medical staffs to organize and implement a quality assurance program that meets the needs of the individual hospital. With a multidisciplinary approach to the quality assurance program, a hospital can develop and implement a comprehensive, problem-focused system that improves the quality of its patient care and clinical performance.

Components of a Quality Assurance Plan

An article by Charles Morris, M.D., director of medical affairs, St. Paul Hospital, Dallas, which appeared in the December 1980 issue of *The Hospital Medical Staff,* cites the nine basic components of a hospitalwide quality assurance plan:

1. **The statement of purpose** states that the board of trustees of the institution is responsible for the development of a medical care evaluation plan. The plan should objectively demonstrate periodic assessment of the quality of medical care and other hospital services and should show that identified deficiencies are actively remedied.

2. **The list of objectives** describes what the plan is intended to achieve, at what level, and under what circumstances.

3. **The statement of authority** identifies which individuals or groups have been delegated responsibility and accountability for implementing the plan. Generally, this delineation of responsibilities defines the obligations of the institution's medical staff, who act under the direction of the board of trustees.

4. **A definition of scope** must be provided. In order to comply with the new JCAH standard, the program must be hospitalwide, comprehensive, and integrated. The size, nature, and complexity of the institution determines the scope of its program.

5. **The organization chart** shows the chain of command and the responsibilities of various persons and groups within the institution. In many institutions, the various responsibilities will be assigned to existing committees that already conduct quality assurance audits.

6. **The statement on how progress and results are reported** should include the titles of those responsible for collecting, collating, and distributing reports; the interval between reports; corrective actions recommended; and an ongoing monitoring plan.
7. **The documentation** and tabulations must be in a form that physicians and other hospital personnel can easily interpret.
8. **The statement on evaluation** helps to determine the effectiveness of the plan in meeting the listed objectives.
9. **The plan for implementing the program** should include a phase-in schedule that will permit a gradual transition from current quality assurance activities to total adoption of the new comprehensive, integrated plan. Although large, complex facilities may require considerable time to make a complete transition, small hospitals should encounter little difficulty.

Operation of a Quality Assurance Plan

After defining the components of a quality assurance plan, Morris outlines the activities involved in operation of the plan.

First, problems must be identified. The JCAH emphasizes a problem-oriented approach to patient care evaluation studies. The procedures that will be used to identify hospital problems and the individuals who will do so must be selected. Personnel in each major department or service are usually most aware of actual or potential problems within that department or service. A variety of data sources may be used to identify problems. These include risk management incident reports; computer printouts on mortality, complications, and lengths of stay; third-party payer denials; utilization review committee reports, chart deficiencies; and deficiencies cited by JCAH. Other data sources that should be considered are individual case reviews, committee minutes, prescription trends, profile analyses, reviews of laboratory and x-ray reports, bylaws infractions, and financial data.

Next, says Morris, a means of selecting problems for study and the rationale used for prioritization must be developed. A quality assurance committee or some comparable multidisciplinary body will usually assume these responsibilities and will assign each study to a responsible individual or department.

The problems that have been identified and chosen for study may be investigated by a retrospective audit, a prospective study, or a concurrent assessment. Regardless of the kind of study that is done, a procedure must be outlined. Such an outline should include a description of criteria development, data gathering procedures, and analysis and display of the study results. A representative of the appropriate department or service may work with the health record analyst (or comparable individual) to develop screening criteria for the study. In a study of a major department, these criteria may be presented to department members for review, critique,

73

comment, revision, and final approval. The scope and time frame of the study also should be included.

Depending on the complexity of the study, individuals in the departments or services studied can be trained to retrieve data. The accumulated data must be analyzed and displayed in such a way that interested individuals can assess its significance.

The quality assurance coordinating function usually reviews the study display to identify the cause and the seriousness of the problem. If the committee determines that corrective action should be taken, the head of the department or service will be asked to suggest solutions. These solutions may include changes in policies or procedures, requests for new equipment, educational endeavors, disciplinary action, or recruitment of more or better qualified personnel. A timetable should be set up to indicate the estimated time required to institute corrective action and to solve the problem.

Most problems studies under the plan can be solved by one-time corrective action. However, if there are chronic problems, it may be necessary to implement a monitoring plan to ensure that the problem does not recur.

Morris points out that each department or service is responsible for documenting the effectiveness of its quality assurance activities and for reporting such activities to the parent committee on a quarterly basis. The quality assurance coordinating function should, in turn, be responsible for documenting that the overall hospital program is functional and effective. The data must be consolidated and reported to the medical staff and to the hospital board of trustees. Such a report might include a description of the problem, the method used to identify the problem, the department or service involved, the person who was assigned to perform the study, the data sources that were used, the cause of the problem, any corrective action that was taken, the person who implemented the action, the timetable for implementation, whether or not the problem was solved, plans for a monitoring procedure, and plans for restudy. Persons involved must remember that quality assurance activities are confidential matters, and special procedures should be followed to avoid or minimize possible incrimination of the parties involved.

Last, the project should be summarized, emphasizing problem identification, problem selection, data retrieval, evaluation, corrective action, resolution, and continual monitoring.

Quality assurance is a dynamic process in which medical record practitioners can work with other hospital personnel and the medical staff in developing, implementing, and maintaining the most effective quality assurance program for the individual.

Quality Assurance in the Medical Record Department

In the same way that a hospital attempts to improve the quality of its services through a hospitalwide quality assurance program, the medical record department can also establish a quality assurance program to improve the quality of its services. A quality assurance program for the medical record department contains the same basic steps as the quality assurance program for the entire hospital. The medical record practitioner must assess current department activities to determine how they would interact with a quality assurance program.

A medical record department quality assurance program should include selection of the topic, medical record department policy, procedure, and so forth that are to be evaluated; development of evaluation criteria or standards; collection of data; analysis of the results; determination of the causes of the variation or problems identified; development and implementation of corrective action; follow-up on the corrective action taken; and reports to administration, medical record department staff, and others.

The department director and staff must develop the objectives for quality assurance activities as well as set standards so that objective review of the activity can take place. Standards can be qualitative or quantitative, and they can be determined through work sampling, direct time studies, or published staffing methodologies.

After the standards for an activity have been set, procedures must be developed to measure the actual practice in the department against the established standards. This measurement will disclose whether department practices meet established standards or whether there are variations or problems in specific areas. If variations or problems exist, the cause as well as corrective steps must be determined. Individuals responsible for corrective action must be clearly identified. Follow-up, at a later date, will provide information on the effectiveness of the corrective action taken.

In the implementation of a quality assurance program, employee orientation to the quality assurance approach to problems and inclusion of employees in the development of standards for their own activities are important. Setting objectives and standards and conducting ongoing evaluations require a time commitment from the department director and staff, and the department director must plan for the cost of implementing a quality assurance program in the department. Ideally, the savings that result from the program will outweigh the initial cost of its establishment.

A medical record department with a quality assurance program will be in compliance with the JCAH requirement, as stated in the *Accreditation Manual for Hospitals:* "The types of data collected and systems of collection within the hospital require internal quality control measures to assess the proficiency of personnel responsible for abstracting and coding medical record information. Verification checks for accuracy, consistency, and uniformity of data recorded and coded for indexes, for statistical record systems, and for use in quality assessment activities should be a regular part of the medical record abstracting process."

The quality assurance program can be used to study internal department operations, such as accuracy of filing in the permanent file; accuracy of the incomplete record locator file; filing of loose material; and accuracy of coding, indexing, and abstracting procedures. By establishing standards for activities and by then measuring current employee activity against these standards, a quality assurance program is an excellent cost containment tool for improving department operations and improving the quality of services rendered.

Risk Management

Another term, *risk management*, has also become a part of the working vocabulary of medical record practitioners. Risk management is the process of identifying, evaluating, and eliminating or controlling risks that pose safety threats to patients or financial threats to the hospital. A hospital's risk management program should be closely related to its quality assurance program. In a hospital with a risk management department, a financial and statistical approach is used, focusing on the patient, nurse, physician, other health care professionals, and ancillary employees. A hospital may employ a risk manager, who evaluates the interaction of all risk components and assesses the risks for the hospital.

For a risk management program to operate successfully, the hospital administration must make a commitment to the program so that the risk manager can become involved in all areas of the hospital that may constitute risks, such as incident reports, employee accidents, and so forth.

The medical record practitioner can assist the risk manager in identifying, evaluating, and eliminating or controlling risks and becomes involved in risk management programs because the medical record is an important screening tool for identifying information relating to hospital risks. The hospital may choose a formal approach to record screening, such as a generic screening for potential patient injury situations, or it may choose to design its own internal system for identifying risks from the medical record.

Utilization Review

The JCAH requires that hospitals have a utilization review program. This program must address overutilization and underutilization within the hospital as well as efficiency in scheduling of resources. JCAH standards list specific requirements for the utilization review plan. Concurrent review and discharge planning are required regardless of the patient's financial status. Nursing and social services may be involved in the preparations for discharge planning.

The utilization review plan should identify the instances in which nonphysician health care professionals may participate in the utilization process. The plan should be reviewed annually and revised when appropriate.

The medical record department is often involved in concurrent reviews and in reviews and initial screenings of patient records at admission and at designated continued-stay review dates. Using written, measurable criteria, and length-of-stay norms that have been approved by the medical staff, medical record practitioners can perform the initial screening of inpatients for the hospital's utilization review plan.

Chapter 10

Statistics

Hospitals generate health care data to satisfy their needs for internal information and to meet the increasing requirements and demands imposed by data users outside the hospital. Detailed data on a broad range of subjects are required for making decisions on utilization management, quality of patient care, cost-containment, payment systems, and so forth.

Traditionally, hospitals have maintained aggregate data on the total numbers of inpatient admissions and discharges, live births, fetal and neonatal deaths, maternal and other deaths, autopsies performed, cesarean sections, nosocomial infections, consultations given, postoperative deaths, surgical operations, and the like. From these data, rates such as average length of stay, occupancy, death, and so forth, were established.

There are many types of health care data and they are useful in a variety of applications. Patient care within hospitals can best be evaluated and managed when adequate information about a large number of inpatients and ambulatory care patients and their treatment is available. Information about not only length of stay, but also about diagnoses, therapies, tests, case outcomes, and procedures can be aggregated and analyzed to gauge the quality, effectiveness, and appropriateness of care rendered to patients in hospitals and by health care professionals. At the national level, the incidence and types of illness and disability, life expectancy, and mortality rates are described by population-based statistics. Health care resources, including the supply of personnel, facilities, and services, can be described statistically. Resource statistics may be related to utilization statistics covering inpatient services, ambulatory care, and types of practices providing services. Information on health care costs, financing, and sources of expenditures are useful in an increasing variety of analyses.

Uniform Hospital Discharge Data Set

The rapid growth in computer capabilities has made possible linkage of data from various sources. However, the problem of definitional differences by providers and users of data has often precluded meaningful comparisons. One of the first steps in identifying, defining, and uniformly recording health care data took place in 1969 when the National Center for Health Statistics and the Johns Hopkins University sponsored a Conference on Hospital Discharge Abstract Systems. The end result of this conference was the development and implementation of the Uniform Hospital Discharge Data Set (UHDDS) to serve as a minimum basic data set for reporting by all short-term general hospitals. In 1974, the Department of Health, Education, and Welfare adopted the UHDDS as departmental policy regarding Medicaid programs and their patient populations. The UHDDS was reviewed and updated in 1980. Conferences have also been held on minimum basic data sets for ambulatory care and long-term care facilities; however, these data sets have not been made final for reporting use.

The UHDDS comprises 14 data items:

- Personal identification, which includes the medical record number and Social Security number on Medicare patients and recipient number on Medicaid patients
- Date of birth
- Sex
- Race and ethnicity
- Residence, specified by zip code
- Hospital identification number
- Admission date
- Discharge date
- Identification of attending physician
- Identification of any operating physician
- Principal diagnosis and other diagnoses
- Significant procedure(s) and date(s)
- Disposition of patient
- Expected principal source of payment

Procedures are reported in accordance with the UHDDS Classes of Procedures for *ICD-9-CM* Procedure Classification. *ICD-9-CM* procedure codes have been grouped into Class 1, 2, 3, or 4 based on procedural risk, anesthetic risk, highly trained personnel required, special facilities required, and special equipment required. It is the responsibility of the medical record practitioner to know and be guided by UHDDS in meeting reporting requirements.

The number and type of patients cared for by a hospital is commonly referred to as its case mix. Research is still being conducted on the best way to determine case mix. Several approaches for describing case mix have been advanced, including diagnosis-related groups (DRGs), disease-staging groups, severity of illness, and type of patient management required. Presently, DRGs are in use in payment systems and utilization review. DRGs are derived from collapsing *ICD-9-CM* codes into a manageable number based on similarity of care or treatment required, using *ICD-9-CM* codes and UHDDS for principal diagnosis, complications, comorbidity, and Class 1, 2, and 3 procedure, and using UHDDS items for age and for disposition.

Data Management

The role of the medical record department has changed dramatically under the Medicare prospective pricing system. Historically, the hospital has been paid on the basis of the patient's length of stay and services rendered, information that was easily obtainable from various sources within the hospital. The new payment system, however, is based on the patient's DRG, which must be assigned according to the documentation in the medical record. Under prospective pricing, the primary function of the medical record director is data management: ensuring that complete, timely, and accurate data are available for DRG assignment and billing purposes. The hospital cannot generate a bill and be paid until the record is complete. Late records, incorrect coding of diagnoses or procedures, or misinterpretation of the record content can lead to underpricing of a patient's stay. Thus, the new role of the medical record department is pivotal to the hospital's finances. The size, skills, and performance levels of medical record staff must be assessed against the requirements of Medicare prospective pricing.

Also, the JCAH *Accreditation Manual for Hospitals* states: "The types of data collected and systems of collection within the hospital require internal quality control measures to assess the proficiency of personnel responsible for abstracting and coding medical record information. Verification checks for accuracy, consistency, and uniformity of data recorded and coded for indexes, for statistical record systems and for use in quality assessment activities should be a regular part of the medical record abstracting process."

Descriptive Statistics

There is increasing emphasis on standardization of health statistics for valid comparisons and analysis. The preferred method is to define a hospital service as a "care unit" according to assigned beds so that assigning units by hospital location is an effective and consistent method of service activity assessment. The more consistently medical record practitioners use standard terminology and reporting methods, the more valid and reliable the results will be.

The following terminology is consistent with the *Glossary of Hospital Terms* of the American Medical Record Association:

Inpatient census. The number of inpatients present at any one time. Example: There are 224 patients in the hospital at 12 midnight.

Inpatient service days. A unit of measure denoting the services received by one inpatient in one 24-hour period. Example: Yesterday the hospital rendered 230 inpatient service days of care.

Daily inpatient census. The number of inpatients present at the census-taking each day plus any inpatients who were both admitted and discharged after the census-taking time the previous day. Example: Yesterday the hospital rendered care to 225 inpatients and 5 patients who were both admitted and discharged during the 24-hour period since the previous day's tally was taken. Therefore, the daily inpatient census was 230.

Length of stay. The number of calendar days from admission to discharge. Example: The patient stayed 5 days.

Discharge days per total length of stay. The sum of the days stay of any group of inpatients discharged during a specified period. Example: The total length of stay for 1540 patients was 540 days.

Other accepted hospital definitions for statistical purposes include hospital patient, hospital inpatient, hospital newborn inpatient, medical staff unit, medical care unit, special care unit, adjunct diagnostic or therapeutic unit, occasion of service, hospital outpatient, emergency outpatient unit, and encounter. These and other terms related to hospital statistics are defined in AMRA's *Glossary of Hospital Terms* and the American Hospital Association's Instructions and Definitions for Annual Survey of Hospitals. *Medical Record Management,* by Edna K. Huffman, published by AMRA, is another useful reference source, especially for sample forms.

In some hospitals, daily census reports are kept according to organized clinical service as well as nursing unit (bed location). Thus, for each service the daily statistical report will show the number of patients admitted directly or by transfer and the number of inpatient service days.

The data gathered should be reviewed periodically so that obsolete material can be discarded and new material added. Since the hospital administration sets the pattern for data collection, medical record personnel should be aware of needs for new data related to activities newly developed in the hospital. Because needs for statistics can change, medical record systems should be organized for flexibility.

Some hospitals gather certain statistics for which there is no general agreement on definition. These data will therefore be useful only to those particular hospitals and to persons who are aware of the limitations of the definitions. Such data may be useful for internal operational purposes.

Hospital Rates

Following are some sample statistical computations of selected hospital rates and ratios. A basic principle of all the rate formulas is the concept of actual versus possible. The number of times an event actually occurred is the numerator of the fraction, and the number of times an event possibly could have occurred is the denominator.

In addition to the rates shown below, hospitals will need to collect more detailed information to complete various reports of agencies such as the JCAH and the AHA. The AHA requests member and nonmember hospitals to complete its Annual Survey of Hospitals. This form requests information on facilities and services, beds and utilization by inpatient service, total hospital beds and utilization, financial data, and information on personnel. The data, with exception of the confidential data, are forwarded to the National Center for Health Statistics for use in updating its inventory of all health care facilities. By using the data, the center does not need to duplicate collection of data from hospitals participating in the survey.

Neonatal death rate

$$= \frac{\text{number of newborn deaths}}{\text{number of newborn discharges, including deaths}} \times 100$$

Example:
$$\frac{4 \text{ newborn deaths}}{431 \text{ newborn discharges}} \times 100 = .93\%$$

Fetal death rate

$$= \frac{\text{number of intermediate and late fetal deaths}}{\begin{array}{c}\text{number of births, including}\\ \text{intermediate and late fetal deaths}\end{array}} \times 100$$

Example:
$$\frac{3 \text{ intermediate/late fetal deaths}}{300 \text{ births}} \times 100 = 1.0\%$$

Cesarean section rate

$$= \frac{\text{number of cesarean sections performed}}{\text{number of deliveries}} \times 100$$

Example:
$$\frac{4 \text{ cesarean sections}}{200 \text{ deliveries}} \times 100 = 2.0\%$$

Average length of stay

$$= \frac{\begin{array}{c}\text{length of stay of patients discharged,}\\ \text{including deaths, excluding newborns}\end{array}}{\begin{array}{c}\text{number of discharges, including deaths,}\\ \text{excluding newborns}\end{array}}$$

Example:
$$\frac{2068 \text{ patient days}}{263 \text{ discharges}} = 7.9 \text{ days}$$

Average daily inpatient census

$$= \frac{\text{number of inpatient service days}}{\text{number of days}}$$

Example:

$$\frac{2100 \text{ inpatient days}}{30 \text{ days}} = 70 \text{ inpatients}$$

Inpatient bed occupancy rate

$$= \frac{\text{inpatient service days}}{\text{number of available beds} \times \text{number of days}} \times 100$$

Example:

$$\frac{6975 \text{ patient days}}{250 \text{ beds} \times 31 \text{ days}} \times 100 = 90\%$$

Gross autopsy rate

$$= \frac{\text{number of inpatient autopsies}}{\text{number of inpatient deaths}} \times 100$$

Example:

$$\frac{9 \text{ inpatient autopsies}}{25 \text{ inpatient deaths}} \times 100 = 36.0\%$$

Net autopsy rate

$$= \frac{\text{number of inpatient autopsies}}{\text{inpatient deaths} - \text{unautopsied coroner or medical examiner cases}} \times 100$$

Example:

$$\frac{9 \text{ inpatient autopsies}}{25 \text{ inpatient deaths} - 7 \text{ unautopsied coroner's cases}} \times 100 = 50.0\%$$

Adjusted autopsy rate

$$= \frac{\text{number of autopsies performed}}{\text{number of patient deaths whose bodies are available for hospital autopsy}} \times 100$$

Example:

$$\frac{9 \text{ inpatient autopsies}}{25 \text{ inpatient deaths} - 7 \text{ unautopsied coroner's cases} + 2 \text{ emergency room death autopsies}} \times 100 = 45\%$$

Hospitalwide death rate

$$= \frac{\text{number of inpatient deaths}}{\text{number of discharges, including deaths}} \times 100$$

Example:

$$\frac{6 \text{ inpatient deaths}}{320 \text{ discharges}} \times 100 = 1.88\%$$

Maternal death rate

$$= \frac{\text{number of maternal deaths}}{\text{number of maternal discharges, including deaths}} \times 100$$

Example:

$$\frac{2 \text{ maternal deaths}}{150 \text{ maternal discharges}} \times 100 = 1.33\%$$

Vital Records

Medical records are the source documents for much of the information needed for birth, death, and fetal death registration certificates, which are used for the state's vital record system. The medical record department may be given the responsibility for preparing birth and fetal death certificates and for transmitting the information to the registrar of vital records.

Medical record personnel must be aware of the importance of prompt and accurate completion of these legal forms. Patient identification data and medical certification information on death certificates are completed by the hospital and attending physicians, and the rest of the information is completed by the mortician. Copies or work sheets of these forms are kept in the medical records for future reference. Every medical record department should have handbooks for registration of births, deaths, and fetal deaths. These can be obtained from the registrar of vital records in the state health department or from the Government Printing Office.

Different states have different regulations regarding vital records. Medical record practitioners must be completely familiar with the regulations in their states so that correct procedures are used. The National Center for Health Statistics, U.S. Public Health Service, Department of Health and Human Services, prepares standard birth, fetal death, and death certificates, which serve as models for use by individual states. Some states require the hospital to maintain a register of births and deaths. This provides readily accessible information without need to refer to patient medical records.

Chapter 11

Preservation of Medical Records

The length of time medical records should be kept and the format in which they should be retained (original or microfilm) are complex issues. In selecting the retention program most consistent with the hospital's operation, the hospital must be guided by its own needs and by existing state laws and potential litigation.

Record Retention

The American Hospital Association's statement *Preservation of Medical Records in Health Care Institutions* was prepared by AHA's Committee on Medical Records in conjunction with the American Medical Record Association's Planning and Bylaws Committee as a step toward promoting uniformity in state laws and regulations relating to statutes of limitation for the retention of medical records. The statement, which was approved by AMRA in 1973 and by AHA in 1974, follows:

The primary purpose of the medical record is to document the course of the patient's illness and the treatment he receives. Although the medical record is kept for the benefit of the patient, the physician, and the health care institution, it is the property of the health care institution with other interests recognized by law.

The length of the time medical records should be retained will vary depending on the purposes for which the record is being kept. In formulating a record retention policy, a health care institution must be guided by its own clinical, scientific, and audit needs, and the possibility of future patient litigation.

In some jurisdictions a health care institution is not required by law to preserve its records for any given length of time. The appropriate period of retention may be affected by the statute of limitations for bringing a legal action for an injury or breach of contract. In most states the period of the applicable statute of limitations would be less than 10 years. Moreover, in many states the statute of limitations requires that an action for personal injuries sustained by a minor must be exercised within a few years after he attains his majority.

It is deemed unnecessary for a health care institution to preserve medical records that duplicate other official records that will be kept permanently. Thus, keeping records for the sole purpose of proving birth or age, residence, citizenship, or family relationship serves no useful purpose. Inasmuch as a hospital or other health care institution is seldom requested to produce medical records older than 10 years for clinical, scientific, legal, or audit purposes, it is ordinarily sufficient to retain the medical records 10 years after the most recent patient care usage in the absence of legal considerations.

Accordingly, it is recommended that complete patient medical records in health care institutions usually be retained, either in the original or reproduced form, for 10 years after the most recent patient care usage. After 10 years, such records may be destroyed unless destruction is specifically prohibited by statute, ordinance, regulation, or law, provided that the institution:

1. Retains basic information such as dates of admission and discharge, names of responsible physicians, records of diagnoses and operations, surgical procedure reports, pathology reports, and discharge resumes for all records so destroyed
2. Retains complete medical records of minors for the period of minority plus the applicable period of statute of limitations as prescribed by statute in the state in which the health care institution is located
3. Retains complete medical records of patients under mental disability in like manner as those of patients under disability of minority
4. Retains complete patient medical records for longer periods when requested in writing by one of the following:
   a. An attending or consultant physician of the patient
   b. The patient or someone acting legally in his behalf
   c. Legal counsel for a party having an interest affected by the patient medical records

If the adoption of a record retention policy as suggested by this statement would reduce the previous period of retention by a health care institution, it is recommended that any new policy be developed with the full knowledge and participation of the medical staff, legal counsel for the institution, and any past or present liability insurance carrier affording coverage during any time in which the affected records were made. It is also recommended that written notice of the new policy of retention be given to state and local medical societies and bar associations and by announcement in any other media suggested by the institution's legal counsel; and, further, that the lesser period of retention either be restricted to subsequently completed patient medical records or the general application be deferred for a reasonable length of time until requests for deferred destruction may be received.

The JCAH states: "The length of time that medical records are to be retained is dependent upon the need for their use in continuing patient care and for legal, research, or educational purposes." The preservation of medical records on a permanent basis may be determined by hospital policy, the statute of limitations or other legal requirements, the foregoing statement of the AHA and AMRA, the needs of the medical staff, and other factors specific to the individual hospital. Medical record practitioners should work with appropriate hospital personnel in developing, implementing, and controlling a retention system that safeguards the physical and information characteristics of medical and health data for future retrieval. Practitioners must carefully consider what types of information to keep, and how long and by what means it is kept.

Microfilming

If the hospital intends to preserve its medical records and does not have space available to keep all records in the paper format, microfilming is an appropriate method of preservation. The terms *microfilm, microform,* or *microimaging* can be applied to any information communication or storage medium containing images too small to be read without magnification. Before microfilming, the medical record department may need to contact the state health department, the hospital licensing agency, or other appropriate state regulatory agency concerning regulations affecting retention of hospital medical records, microfilming requirements, and specific provisions accompanying microfilm permissibility as evidence in court. The hospital attorney should also be consulted in decisions involving microfilming. This individual will be aware of specific microfilming regulations affecting operations in that particular state. Some states require authorization or approval from the regulatory agency before the original records may be destroyed. The department needs to be familiar with any legal ramifications regarding microfilming and future use of the film. If space is critical, the hospital may be able to obtain permission to microfilm records earlier than state regulation permits.

The hospital can elect to microfilm entirely inhouse with hospital personnel, to contract with an outside company, or to use a combination of the above. For example, the hospital could choose to do chart preparation using hospital personnel with the actual microfilming done by the service company. Regardless of the plan selected, the original medical records should not be destroyed until medical record or other personnel designated by the hospital have reviewed the microfilm for quality of film production and for accuracy in microfilming.

If the hospital chooses to contract for its microfilming needs with a microfilm service bureau, which is usually a private business that provides micrographic services using a customer's own material, the hospital should consider the following:

- Range of services offered
- Type or condition of equipment used
- Staff expertise
- Record of performance in similar applications
- Understanding of application requirements
- Ability to provide high-quality services within the time allotted
- Cost
- Availability of service in the local area

Microfilming can be done annually, semiannually, or quarterly. If space needs are acute and if records are microfilmed within three to five years following dismissal of the patients, a quarterly schedule may be desirable. The activity of the records is the key factor in determining the retention and microfilming schedule. The hospital may choose to retire old records at the same rate new records enter the system.

Microfilm storage and retrieval systems are designed to enable users to locate a desired image from among thousands of images. The hospital can select from various methods and media to house the microfilm, as follows.

Roll film, which may contain several hundred charts on each roll, may be suitable for serially numbered records, provided requests for past records are few. Roll film is the most economical media. Its major disadvantage is that the confidentiality of other patients may be jeopardized if a particular record is requested in court and the entire roll is submitted.

Cartridges and cassettes are designed for users who want the advantages of roll microfilm without the inconvenience of the manual film handling. Cartridges and cassettes offer more flexibility and consequently are more expensive than roll film.

Microfiche, which is a sheet of film containing multiple microimages, has the advantage of easy and direct access to information, because all the information on a patient appears on an individual sheet. Some microfiche can be updated, a feature that allows information microfilmed later to be housed with the original record. Microfilm jackets of transparent acetate can be used to hold microfilm in flat strips. New images can be added to the jacket or old images deleted.

Computer output microfilm (COM) is a process by which digital data are converted to readable text or graphic information in microfilm without first creating paper documents. The computer creates magnetic tapes that contain data for generating reports. COM has applications in computerizing a master patient index as well as other applications.

Overall, the hospital needs an effective retention and retrieval program to access information for research, statistics, and educational purposes. The medical record department must be able to provide accurate, complete, and useful data from patient records after discharge and is responsible for providing this information in the most effective manner possible.

Guidelines on Institutional Policies for Disclosure of Medical Record Information

These guidelines were developed by the American Hospital Association's Advisory Panel on Privacy and Confidentiality of Hospital Medical Records to promote and preserve the confidentiality of hospital medical records and to establish principles and recommendations for appropriate access to them. These guidelines were approved by the AHA Board of Trustees in November 1978.

Introduction

Changes in the social and economic environment, accompanied by rapid growth in record-keeping capabilities, have produced an intensive need and demand for more kinds of and more detailed patient and patient care information. Never before have hospitals had to keep so much information to make possible the completion of daily transactions involving patient care and delivery of services. Never before have hospital medical records been subjected to so many demands for their use and disclosure of contents.

The informational upsurge is largely the result of:

- Increasing complexity of medical care associated with the growth in size and variety of professional disciplines involved in the delivery of health care services.
- Wide-scale use of computers in marshaling information, processing information exchange, and creating data banks.
- Increasing mobility of the population, with the consequent increase in the volume of requests for exchange of medical information.
- Expanding informational needs of governmental agencies for planning, administration, evaluation of government programs, and policymaking purposes.

- Progressive growth in the number of third parties* concerned with the patient and his medical record. Many of these third parties are seeking information for proposed uses, such as payment for patient care, that are quite different from the primary purpose for which it was collected.
- Increased government access to patient-identifiable records and increased reporting of personal information to the government.
- Increased incidence of health-related legal actions and proceedings.
- Potential misuse of the authorization for disclosure of medical record information.

A searching examination by the American Hospital Association on how best to use and control hospital medical records brought forth contrasting and sometimes conflicting views on how to ensure privacy rights while at the same time recognizing the legitimate interests of third parties. Of concern to the Association is the prevailing tendency of information seekers to disregard or be unaware of the hospital's obligation to respect the right of patients to personal privacy and to treat records pertaining to their care as confidential.

As the first step in striking a proper balance between the personal privacy rights of patients and the informational needs of hospitals and society in general, the American Hospital Association believes that it is essential for hospitals to have a well-defined policy on the use and disclosure of medical information. This policy should limit disclosures to essential purposes, restrict information disclosure to that necessary to accomplish those essential purposes, promote the use of an authorization for disclosure of medical records, and recognize the limitations of the medical record in performing the many services expected of it. However, provision should be made for those instances when nothing less than a full disclosure of the medical record will suffice.

These guidelines have been prepared to assist hospitals in developing policy manuals on the disclosure of medical record information. Following the concepts of policy formation, the guidelines define areas in which decisions are made and establish policies to cover the areas deemed important. Principles established for internal use differ from those established for external use. Recognition also is given to the exceptional situations that may require special handling.

Characteristics of the Medical Record

The development of policies on disclosure of medical record content must begin with a set of basic principles. These basic principles relate to the

---

*A party other than the patient, the patient's personal representative, the physician, or the hospital.

characteristics of the medical record: purpose, content and format, disclosure, ownership, confidentiality, and accessibility of the medical record.

Purpose

The primary purpose of the medical record is to document the course of the patient's illness and treatment during all periods of care, whether as an inpatient or outpatient. The record is important in medical practice. It serves as an instrument for communication among physicians and other professionals contributing to the patient's care and as a basis for planning and evaluating that care. The secondary purposes of the medical record are:

- To serve as a source for substantiation of the patient care services and treatment provided
- To provide clinical data of interest to researchers and continuing education programs
- To meet and support legal and quasi-legal obligations imposed on the hospital and the physician

Content and Format

The medical record is used by practitioners in the management of patient care. Because of this use, the objectives of effective patient care should serve as the basis for determining content, methods of organizing clinical information, desired manner and style of recording, adequacy and timeliness of entries, and justification for exclusion or inclusion of information.

Ownership

Records of the hospital, including medical records maintained for the benefit of the patient, the physician, and the hospital, are regarded as the property of the hospital. Legal counsel should be consulted as to applications of local laws.

Disclosure

Subject to applicable legal provisions, the hospital may restrict removal of medical records from its files or from its premises, determine who may have access to their contents, and define the information that may be disclosed. In fact, state laws or regulations, or the need to preserve the admissibility of records as evidence in judicial proceedings, may mandate that records be removed only for hospital or courtroom purposes.

Confidentiality

The patient has the right to expect that records pertaining to his care will be treated as confidential, and the hospital has the obligation to safeguard his records against unauthorized disclosure.

Accessibility

Medical records should be used within the hospital only by authorized recipients on a need-to-know basis. Responsibility for disclosure of medical record information by the hospital, with or without the authorization of the patient to whom it pertains, should be delegated to hospital personnel who understand the characteristics of the medical record and recognize the occasional situations that require the advice of a medical staff member or the hospital attorney.

Policies for Internal Disclosure

The hospital shall provide for the security of the medical record and establish internal policies to provide for their proper use as needed to carry out functions within the hospital. Access to the medical record without the written consent of the patient depends on:

- The authority and responsibility of the hospital or medical staff member or duly appointed committee or panel requesting access
- The reason for the request
- The kind of information required

Policies for internal disclosure of medical record information should be established for various functions within the hospital as described in the following paragraphs.

Governing Board and Chief Executive Officer

Legal precedents recognize the right of access by the governing board of the hospital in order to ensure quality of patient care. All hospital policies on the use of the medical record and on disclosure of medical record content should be prepared in consultation with the hospital attorney and are subject to review by the governing board of the hospital.

The chief executive officer has access to all records of patients whenever necessary to carry out his management responsibility. Except when laws or regulations dictate otherwise, the chief executive officer also has the responsibility for final decisions on what medical record disclosures may be made and the circumstances under which disclosures may be made.

Hospital Security

It is the responsibility of the hospital to establish and implement security measures that reasonably safeguard both the medical record and its informational content, whether in hard copy, on film, or in computerized form, against loss, defacement, tampering, unauthorized disclosure, and use by unauthorized persons. All officers and employees of the hospital must be made aware of their responsibility in maintaining the confidentiality of medical record information and of the disciplinary actions that may be taken for unauthorized disclosures of patient-identifiable information.

Patient Care

Use of a patient's previous medical record, both inpatient and outpatient, by physicians and other health care professionals involved in the care of that patient at the institution maintaining the record does not require the patient's signed authorization because consent to such use is implied. Disclosure of medical information in the event of direct referral or transfer of the patient to another medical care provider does not require the patient's signed authorization. A record should be kept of the information disclosed.

Quality Evaluation

Because of its responsibility for determining whether the quality of care provided to all patients is consistent with standards as provided for in the medical staff bylaws and in the requisites for hospital accreditation, the hospital can use medical record information for quality evaluation without the express authorization of the individual patient to whom it pertains. However, all individual patient identification should be excluded from the routine report of such findings and recommendations. When circumstances dictate otherwise, a coded method of identification may be appropriate for internal use.

Education Programs

The hospital should establish rules for the use of medical records in hospital-approved education programs for medical and health care professions and should disseminate the rules to the appropriate program directors and instructors, who also must share the responsibility for protecting the confidentiality of the medical records and ensuring the availability of the records for patient care purposes.

Research

The rules of the hospital shall define the extent to which physicians and other health care professional staff in good standing are privileged to use the medical records for bona fide study and research and shall define circumstances that require patient authorization for such use. Anyone using the medical records for bona fide study and research must also share the responsibility for protecting the confidentiality of the medical records and ensuring the availability of the records for patient care purposes.

Health Data Systems and Data Registries*

The hospital, as a provider and user of data resulting from its maintenance of and/or participation in a health data system, shall ensure that reasonable care is taken to:

---

*For further information, see the AHA Statement on Health Care Data, AHA catalog no. 097732.

- Safeguard the privacy rights of persons identified therein
- Collect and store relevant information
- Establish standards for accuracy, timeliness, and completeness of data input
- Obtain and maintain security of confidential data
- Control unauthorized disclosure in patient-identifiable, physician-identifiable, or hospital-identifiable form
- Validate statistical data
- Closely monitor the data system for its continuing adherence to previously agreed upon policies and procedures

Hospital Affairs

Access to the medical record without patient authorization should be provided only on a need-to-know basis in the management of hospital affairs, including that necessary for performing internal administrative tasks, conducting quality assurance programs, receiving legal counsel, planning health services, and surveying hospital-approved programs for accreditation compliance. Staff access to medical records shall be commensurate with a person's responsibility and authority for conducting hospital business. Disclosures of medical record content shall be made only by those suitably trained or qualified to do so.

Policies for External Disclosure

The hospital shall establish policies for the disclosure of medical record information to meet the various controls and requests that arise from outside the hospital. Elements to be considered in policy formulation include:

- Types of requests
- Kind of information requested
- Persons, agencies, or organizations authorized to receive information
- Permission needed for disclosure
- Conformance to laws, regulations, and other measures in the public interest
- Establishment of reasonable charges for furnishing copies

Provision should be made for handling exceptional requests that result in decisions that may constitute additional policies or important modifications of existing policies.

Policies for external disclosure should be established to cover all events usually faced by the hospital as described below.

Authorization for Disclosure

The hospital shall respect each patient's expectation that records pertaining to his care will be treated as confidential. Therefore, no hospital should disclose, or be required to disclose, medical record information in patient-identifiable form to a third party without the patient's authorization, unless such disclosure is:

- Pursuant to law or statutory regulations requiring the hospital to report certain information
- In accordance with compelling circumstances affecting a person's health or safety
- Permitted under certain circumstances by the hospital in the conduct of biomedical, epidemiologic, or health services research projects
- Limited to name, date of admission, and general condition, except in those instances when the patient or his authorized representative requests that even this limited information not be released or when laws or regulations (for example, alcohol and drug abuse treatment) forbid the disclosure of this information

Patient Authorization

Written authorizations are a good practice and may be mandated under some regulatory requirements; for example, the Federal Drug and Alcohol Abuse Act.

One of the purposes of a well-drawn authorization for disclosure of medical record information is to indicate to the patient, or person acting on his behalf, what subject matter is being authorized to be disclosed, the person or organization that will receive the information, and any applicable time limit (see pages 107 to 109).

Disclosure Limits

The hospital has a responsibility to limit the disclosure of information to only that which is stated on the authorization or required by law and to limit disclosures made without the patient's authorization to only that information permitted or required by law to accomplish the purpose for which the disclosure is made. Whenever disclosure is made pursuant to the written consent of a patient involved in a drug or alcohol abuse program or treatment function, such disclosure must be accompanied by the following statement: "This information has been disclosed to you from records whose confidentiality is protected by Federal law. Federal regulations prohibit you from making any further redisclosure of it without the specific written consent of the person to whom it pertains."

Record of Authorization

The hospital should maintain either the original or copies of the patient's disclosure authorization, which should be made available for examination by the patient.

Careful consideration should be given to keeping a notation of all disclosures to third parties.

Other Health Care Providers

The hospital shall not honor a request from another hospital, a nonstaff physician, or other health care provider for patient-identifiable medical record information unless the request is accompanied by that patient's authorization for disclosure, except under certain conditions warranting immediate disclosure to a properly identified medical care provider or public health officer. Examples are: (1) a showing of compelling circumstances affecting the health or safety of a person or (2) when needed in connection with a direct referral or transfer of the patient from the hospital to another medical care provider.

Third-Party Contractors

The hospital shall not disclose, without the patient's authorization, information from the patient's medical record pursuant to the hospital's agreement with a government agency or other third-party payer for payment of hospital service charges to authorized beneficiaries or clients of such a program or plan, unless disclosure is:

- Granted by the hospital on behalf of a patient to determine benefits entitlement when the patient is unable to communicate an authorization for disclosure
- In accordance with provisions of a particular hospital / third-party agreement for inspection of certain portions of a medical record in the performance of claims processing or financial audit

Insurance Carriers

The hospital shall not disclose to an insurance company or insurance plan any patient-identifiable medical record information maintained by the hospital unless the request is accompanied by the patient's authorization for disclosure or by an authorization for disclosure of information necessary to process the insurance claim(s).

Hospital Accreditation and Licensure Surveys

The hospital shall acknowledge the requisites of hospital accreditation and state licensure bodies to review medical records maintained by the hospital only to the extent required or expressly authorized in the performance of their duties to ensure compliances with approved standards or statutory regulations for medical records, provided the reports of such surveys do not directly or indirectly identify any individual patient.

Government Programs

The hospital shall recognize requests for access to or reports of patient-identifiable medical record information for evaluation, audit, or certification purposes by government agencies pursuant to the administration of a government program only to the extent expressly authorized in applicable statues or regulations, or if the hospital receives an administrative summons expressly authorized in applicable statutes and issued by administrative or executive authority of government or a judicial subpoena or court order. The summons should identify particular record(s) and / or items of information to be made available to the agency.

Evidence and Investigation

The hospital should disclose to attorneys, tribunals, members of the court, or government investigation and law enforcement agencies medical record information in patient-identifiable form only if disclosure is authorized by the patient, unless disclosure is compelled by judicial subpoena, court order, properly issued and authorized administrative summons, or as otherwise mandated by law.

Biomedical, Epidemiologic, or Health Services Research

The hospital's chief executive officer shall determine whether or not to permit medical records maintained by the hospital to be used by a third party for purposes of conducting biomedical, epidemiologic, health services, or related research and whether or not the patient's authorization is required in accordance with established hospital policy.

The following determinants should be considered in making the decision:

- The importance of the project's purpose outweighs any nominal risk to individual privacy rights
- The proposed methodology does not violate any limitations under which the medical record information was collected
- The safeguards are adequate to protect the confidentiality and integrity of the medical record and information therein
- The further use or redisclosure of any medical record information in patient-identifiable, physician-identifiable, or hospital-identifiable form requires the written consent of the chief executive officer of the hospital, who shall exercise due regard for the rights of others affected
- The medical records of the hospital are a suitable source of information for the purpose for which they are to be used
- The third party makes appropriate commitments for safeguarding the patient's privacy, including, in some instances, an agreement to refrain from contacting the patient or others

Public Health Laws

The hospital should disclose, without patient authorization, medical record information in patient-identifiable form pursuant to the provisions of state vital statistics laws, which mandate registration of birth, deaths, and fetal deaths, and of other public health laws that compel reporting of certain epidemiologic conditions.

School Referrals

The hospital should not disclose to administration personnel, teachers, or nurses in the local school system the results of diagnostic tests on students referred to the hospital by the school system unless such disclosure is authorized by the student's parent(s) or guardian or, if the student is an adult or emancipated minor, by the student.

Employer Requests

The hospital should not disclose to an employer any information on an employee who is the subject of a medical record maintained by the hospital without the employee's authorization for disclosure, unless such disclosure is pursuant to any state or local statute(s) providing specific authority for such disclosure.

Policies for Disclosure to Patients

The American Hospital Association's statement entitled *A Patient's Bill of Rights** states: "The patient has the right to obtain from his physician complete current information concerning his diagnosis, treatment, and prognosis in terms the patient can be reasonably expected to understand. When it is not medically advisable to give such information to the patient, the information should be made available to an appropriate person in his behalf."

In addition to information available from the physician, the law (statutory or judicial) of most states recognizes a reasonable right of access to medical record information by the patient or his nominees. The patient's right of access in no way abrogates the hospital's property rights in its record and its right to establish reasonable procedures for access to the patient's record. The attending physician should be notified of the patient's request for access to the medical record. Records containing information that might be detrimental to the physical and / or mental health of the patient, as determined by the attending physician, should be released in a form that minimizes any adverse effect on the patient.

When it is known that patient access to medical record information may be medically contraindicated, the hospital may require that a physician or his designee inspect the record and communicate the appropriate information.

Fairness Protection

The hospital's record-keeping relationship with the patient on whom it maintains a medical record is that of fairness and protection of confidential information.

---

*American Hospital Association. *A Patient's Bill of Rights*. AHA catalog no. 157758. Chicago. 1975.

- A person has the right to verify that the hospital has created and is maintaining a medical record pertaining to care or services provided to the person by the hospital
- A patient has the right to find out that a disclosure of his medical record has been made and to whom it has been made, if such information is available
- A patient has the right to expect the hospital to exercise reasonable care in protecting the confidentiality of the medical records it maintains
- Unless access is believed by the attending physician to be medically contraindicated, the patient may look at the record of medical care provided, may request a copy upon payment of reasonable charges for the service, and may request correction or amendment of information
- A patient's personal representative(s) or duly authorized nominee(s), upon good cause shown by such person(s), may be granted reasonable access to information contained within the patient's medical record

Development of Policy and Procedure

The hospital should develop a policy for internal use that sets forth (1) a person's ability to verify whether or not the hospital maintains a medical record of care and services provided to that person and (2) the scope of a patient's right of reasonable access to the record of medical care provided. The policy should encompass existing centralized and departmentalized systems of medical records. Development of the policy and the related procedures should take into consideration:

- The responsibility of the hospital to provide reasonable administrative, technical, and physical safeguards to ensure that records are disclosed only as expressly specified in applicable laws and regulations, in the patient's signed authorization, and in the hospital's written policies and procedures
- The identification of record systems within the hospital, such as records created and kept on inpatients, outpatients, emergency service patients, home-care patients, and private outpatients referred for diagnostic or therapeutic services
- The delineation of hospital policy and any regulatory requirements on preservation, retention, and retirement schedules for patient-identifiable records, including those collected and maintained within the various departments of the hospital
- Measures to provide evidence of all disclosures of medical record information, other than those made during routine use within the hospital, and the retention of such evidence with the record from which the information was disclosed

- The notification of the attending or responsible physician(s) when a patient requests access to his medical record
- The designation of a committee or a hospital staff member and a medical staff member who are granted authority and responsibility for implementing and overseeing hospital policy and procedures on patient access to medical records and reviewing judgment thereunder
- The steps involved in receiving and considering the patient's request for a correction of or an amendment to this medical record, including notification to the attending or responsible physician of such request and notification to the patient as to the acceptance or denial of the request
- The establishment of a mechanism, which might consist of a committee or panel, to review denial of a patient's request to correct or amend his record
- The establishment of special procedures to handle requests by the patient or the patient's family for access to medical records when direct access apparently could be harmful to the patient
- The identification of a minor's right to access to the medical record as may be permitted under general state law or state law permitting a minor to seek on his own behalf, without the knowledge or consent of his parents, treatment for certain conditions, such as venereal disease, alcohol or drug abuse, and pregnancy, and for family planning and abortion services

However, when a claim against the hospital or its medical staff members is threatened or pending, or after suit has actually been filed, requests by patients or their attorneys or other representatives for access to the patient's medical records should be brought to the hospital attorney's attention immediately. The attorney may then advise whether, when, how, and under what circumstances such access should be granted or copies furnished to the requesters.

If state law permits a minor to obtain certain treatment without the knowledge or consent of his parents, there may be instances in which only the minor may have access to the medical record, or the minor must give consent for his parent(s) or guardian to obtain the information. Hospitals will need legal advice on any provisions related to minors in existing laws, such as in laws concerned with drug or alcohol abuse, venereal disease, certain other contagious diseases, pregnancy, family planning, and abortion.

Suggested Practices for Notification and Access

The relationship of the hospital's medical record-keeping practices to the patient's stated interest in the medical record maintained by the hospital is that of fairness in the procedures developed to:

- Confirm to a person, upon request, whether or not a record of medical care provided is currently kept by the hospital

- Allow a patient to find out, if the information is available, whether or not a patient-identifiable disclosure has been made to a third party and, if so, to whom it was disclosed
- Arrange for a patient to see and / or obtain a copy of the record of medical care provided, or portions thereof, and allow the patient, if so desired, to be accompanied by a person chosen by the patient
- Arrange for access to the medical record by a qualified medical care professional and / or other responsible person so designated by the patient when direct access by the patient is deemed medically contraindicated by the attending physician
- Consider a patient's request for correction or amendment of the medical record and, if not granted, allow a statement of the patient's disagreement to be filed in the record of medical care provided

The hospital should designate a specific office to which all inquiries related to a person's interest in the record of medical care provided, including those received by mail, telephone, or delivered in person, should be referred.

Hospital procedures should be developed to inform persons requesting information about a medical record or access to a record that such requests should be free from ambiguity or uncertainty as to identification of the patient. Such requests for information should:

- Be made in writing, signed, and mailed or delivered to the designated office
- Describe the type(s) or scope of records being sought and the manner of response desired by the inquirer

When identification of a person or the person's designee is uncertain, the inquirer may be asked to give further or more certain identification, such as date of birth, known or approximate dates of visits or admissions to the hospital, and any known hospital identification numbers, such as medical record or account number. Persons who mail, deliver, or complete in person a written request that contains insufficient identifying or other information should be advised of the additional requirements.

Responses to all written requests pertaining to notification or access should be made promptly, if possible within 10 business days following their receipt. If a full response cannot be made within that time, an acknowledgement should be sent to indicate that a response will be forthcoming.

If there is no evidence of an existing record or if the record in question has been retired, the inquirer should be so advised.

If identification is made and the record is available, the attending or responsible physician(s) should be notified of the request.

Form letters may be prepared to:

- Confirm whether the hospital maintains, subject to record retirement policies, a medical record on the person who is the subject of the

inquiry, which may indicate inpatient, outpatient, emergency service care, utilization of only departmental services, or other type of record
- Act as a cover letter accompanying the transmission of requested information to the patient or patient's authorized representative
- Send notices of fees, to be remittted in advance, to cover the routine costs for preparing copies
- Notify when and where the records will be available for personal inspection

Procedures for Personal Access

If a patient elects to see and / or obtain a copy of the record, the attending or responsible physician(s) should be notified and the patient should be informed that:
- The record will be available at a certain place on specified days and during given hours.
- The patient may be required to furnish adequate self-identification.
- If the patient chooses to have another person present during the review, the hospital may require the patient to sign a statement to that effect.

To ensure the integrity of a medical record during such personal review, a designated hospital employee should be present at all times. To the extent feasible or desirable, a physician or qualified employee may be present to assist the patient in reading the entries in the record.

Requests for Correction or Amendment

A patient's request for correction of or amendment to the medical record should be submitted in writing and should specify the entry or entries in dispute. With the exception of requests for correction of such items as time of admission, birthdate, spelling of name, and other such admission data that can be handled by qualified employees, the attending or other responsible physician(s) should be notified of requests received for corrections or amendments. The hospital attending physician(s) will decide whether or not the correction or amendment is to be made.

If the decision is made to correct or amend the record, the patient should be so advised. Any correction or amendment should not obliterate the material corrected.

If the request for correction or amendment is not granted, the patient should be informed that a statement of the patient's disagreement can be filed with the hospital and that the disputed entries in his medical record will be appropriately annotated to reflect this disagreement. Any further disclosure of the medical record will include this statement of disagreement and the annotations.

106

Model Authorization for Disclosure

In determining the effectiveness of an authorization for medical record disclosure, the following elements would be considered necessary under the laws of most states:

- Name or other sufficient designation of the hospital or other custodian of the medical record to which the authorization is addressed.
- Names of each person, firm, corporation, or public body to which information or copies of records may be released by the custodian of medical records.
- Adequate designation of information to be disclosed, subject to restrictions by the patient to disclosure of a specific medical condition, injury, time period, and / or any other type of specified information.
- Signature of the patient on whom the medical record is maintained, or of a person lawfully authorized to act in the patient's behalf, and the date the authorization form was signed.
- Specified expiration date, if consistent with purpose of disclosure. For example, the patient may wish the authorization to be for a reasonable specified time period, except when an authorization is presented in connection with a life or noncancellable or guaranteed renewable health insurance policy or with payment claims for health services provided. In the absence of a contract, an authorization may be revoked by the consenter at any time.
- Agreement by the recipient not to further disclose such information, or make copies of it, unless further disclosure is expressly permitted in the original authorization or is by necessary implication inherent in the purposes of the original consent or authorization.
- Prohibition of proposed new use of information without additional written consent.

Using the desired elements of an authorization for disclosure of medical record information, authorization forms can be developed to provide a reasonable assurance that a patient may authorize disclosure only to the extent desired. A suggested form for this purpose is shown on page 109.

Other and more specialized forms may be devised for special purposes, such as release of information to facilitate payment of hospital services provided. An example of such a form is shown on the next page.

Example of Authorization for Disclosure
of Information for Hospital Payment

Patient's Name _____

Re: Admission or hospital services commencing _____
DATE

The undersigned hereby authorizes _____
NAME OF HEALTH CARE PROVIDER

to release to _____
INSURANCE CARRIER(S) OR NAME OF PARTY THAT IS OR MAY BE LIABLE FOR ALL OR PART OF THE
HOSPITAL CHARGES

_____

only such diagnostic and therapeutic information (including any treatment for alcohol or
drug abuse) as may be necessary to determine benefits entitlement and to process payment
claims for health care services provided to the above named patient.

This authorization shall be valid only for the period of time necessary to actually process
payment claims pertaining to the patient but in any case shall cease to be valid _____
years from this date.

Signature _____ Date _____
IF SIGNED BY PERSONAL REPRESENTATIVE, STATE RELATIONSHIP TO DO SO

ANY DISCLOSURE OF MEDICAL RECORD INFORMATION
BY THE RECIPIENT(S) IS PROHIBITED EXCEPT WHEN IMPLICIT
IN THE PURPOSES OF THIS DISCHARGE

108

Example of Authorization for Disclosure of Medical Record Information

Subject's name: _____ _____
               LAST   FIRST   MIDDLE INITIAL   BIRTHDATE AND AGE

Address: _____ _____
                    STREET, CITY, STATE   PHONE

The undersigned hereby authorizes and requests _____
                                                HEALTH CARE OR HEALTH SERVICES PROVIDER

to provide _____
           IDENTITY OF THIRD PARTY OR NAME(S) OF ANY DULY AUTHORIZED REPRESENTATIVE(S)

_____

with access to my medical / hospital records for the purpose of review and examination and
further authorizes and requests that you provide such copies thereof as may be requested.

The foregoing is subject to such limitation as indicated below:

( ) 1. Confined to records regarding admission and treatment for the following medical
       condition or injury:

       _____

       on or about _____at the following facility:_____
                        DATE

       _____

( ) 2. Covering records for the period from _____ to _____
                                                  DATE   DATE

( ) 3. Confined to the following specified information: _____

       _____

( ) 4. No limitations placed on dates, history of illness, or diagnostic and therapeutic in-
       formation, including any treatment for alcohol and drug abuse. (Signer to initial
       for authentication of this response) _____

Expiration date of this authorization, if any:_____

Signature:_____ Date: _____
          IF SIGNED BY PERSONAL REPRESENTATIVE, STATE RELATIONSHIP AND AUTHORITY TO DO SO

ANY DISCLOSURE OF MEDICAL RECORD INFORMATION
BY THE RECIPIENT(S) IS PROHIBITED EXCEPT WHEN IMPLICIT
IN THE PURPOSES OF THIS DISCLOSURE

114